Contents

Notes on contributors

Yu-Ju Chien   Department of Sociology, University of Minnesota, Minneapolis MN, United States

Robert Dingwall   Dingwall Enterprises and School of Social Sciences, Nottingham Trent University, UK

Muriel Figuié   Centre de coopération internationale en recherche agronomique pour le développement, Montpellier, France

Martin French   Department of Media, Culture and Communication, New York University, United States

Claude Gilbert   CNRS (UMR PACTE), Politique et Organisations, Grenoble, France

Maya K. Gislason   Centre for Global Health Policy, University of Sussex, Brighton

Rebecca Godderis   Health Studies, Wilfrid Laurier University, Brantford, Ontario, Canada

Lily M. Hoffman   Department of Sociology, The City College and Graduate Center, City University of New York, United States.

Colin Jerolmack   Department of Sociology, New York University, United States

Tanya Kolobov   Department of Sociology, University of Haifa, Israel

Erika Mansnerus   LSE Health, London School of Economics and Political Science; and Department of Social Science, Health and Medicine, King's College, London

Sabrina McCormick   Department of Environmental and Occupational Health, George Washington University, Washington DC, United States

Gustavo S. Mesch   Department of Sociology, University of Haifa, Israel

Eric Mykhalovskiy   Department of Sociology, York University, Toronto, ON, Canada

Jocelyn Raude   Department of Social and Behavioural Sciences, EHESP School of Public Health, Rennes, France

Kate Rossiter   Health Studies, Wilfrid Laurier University, Brantford, Ontario, Canada

Kent P. Schwirian   Department of Sociology, The Ohio State University, Columbus, Ohio, United States

William Sherlaw   Department of International Relations, EHESP School of Public Health, Rennes, France

Greg Smith   School of Humanities, Languages and Social Sciences, University of Salford

Karen Staniland   College of Health and Social Care, University of Salford, UK

Véronique Steyer   ISG Paris, GrIIsG, and ESCP Europe, Stratégie, Hommes et Organisations, Paris, France

Rosemary C.R. Taylor   Department of Sociology/Community Health Program, Tufts University, Medford, MA, United States

Kristoffer Whitney   Holtz Center for Science and Technology Studies, University of Wisconsin-Madison, Madison WI, United States

Pandemics and Emerging Infectious Diseases

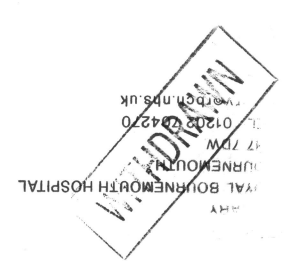

Sociology of Health and Illness Monograph Series

Edited by Professor Ian Rees Jones
Cardiff School of Social Sciences
WISERD
46 Park Place
Cardiff
CF10 3BB
Wales, UK

Current titles

Pandemics and Emerging Infectious Diseases: The Sociological Agenda (2013)
edited by *Robert Dingwall, Lily M. Hoffman and Karen Staniland*

The Sociology of Medical Screening: Critical Perspectives, New Directions (2012)
edited by *Natalie Armstrong and Helen Eborall*

Body Work in Health and Social Care: Critical Themes, New Agendas (2011)
edited by *Julia Twigg, Carol Wolkowitz, Rachel Lara Cohen and Sarah Nettleton*

Technogenarians: Studying Health and Illness Through an Ageing, Science, and Technology Lens (2010)
edited by *Kelly Joyce and MeikaLoe*

Communication in Healthcare Settings: Policy, Participation and New Technologies (2009)
edited by *Alison Pilnick, Jon Hindmarsh and Virginia Teas Gill*

Pharmaceuticals and Society: Critical Discourses and Debates (2009)
edited by *Simon J. Williams, Jonathan Gabe and Peter Davis*

Ethnicity, Health and Health Care: Understanding Diversity, Tackling Disadvantage (2008)
edited by *Waqar I. U. Ahmad and Hannah Bradby*

The View From Here: Bioethics and the Social Sciences (2007)
edited by *Raymond de Vries, Leigh Turner, Kristina Orfali and Charles Bosk*

The Social Organisation of Healthcare Work (2006)
edited by *Davina Allen and Alison Pilnick*

Social Movements in Health (2005)
edited by *Phil Brown and Stephen Zavestoski*

Health and the Media (2004)
edited by *Clive Seale*

Partners in Health, Partners in Crime: Exploring the boundaries of criminology and sociology of health and illness (2003)
edited by *Stefan Timmermans and Jonathan Gabe*

Rationing: Constructed Realities and Professional Practices (2002)
edited by *David Hughes and Donald Light*

Rethinking the Sociology of Mental Health (2000)
edited by *Joan Busfield*

Sociological Perspectives on the New Genetics (1999)
edited by *Peter Conrad and Jonathan Gabe*

The Sociology of Health Inequalities (1998)
edited by *Mel Bartley, David Blane and George Davey Smith*

The Sociology of Medical Science (1997)
edited by *Mary Ann Elston*

Health and the Sociology of Emotion (1996)
edited by *Veronica James and Jonathan Gabe*

Medicine, Health and Risk (1995)
edited by *Jonathan Gabe*

Pandemics and Emerging Infectious Diseases
The Sociological Agenda

Edited by

Robert Dingwall, Lily M. Hoffman
and Karen Staniland

WILEY-BLACKWELL

A John Wiley & Sons, Ltd., Publication

This edition first published 2013
Originally published as Volume 35, Issue 2 of *The Sociology of Health & Illness*
Chapters © 2013The Authors.
Book Compilation © 2013 Foundation for the Sociology of Health & Illness/John Wiley & Sons Ltd.

Registered Office
John Wiley & Sons Ltd, The Atrium, Southern Gate, Chichester, West Sussex, PO19 8SQ, United Kingdom

Editorial Offices
350 Main Street, Malden, MA 02148-5020, USA
9600 Garsington Road, Oxford, OX4 2DQ, UK
The Atrium, Southern Gate, Chichester, West Sussex, PO19 8SQ, UK

For details of our global editorial offices, for customer services, and for information about how to apply for permission to reuse the copyright material in this book please see our website at www.wiley.com/wiley-blackwell.

Library of Congress Cataloging-in-Publication Data

Pandemics and emerging infectious diseases : the sociological agenda / edited by Robert
Dingwall, Lily M. Hoffman and Karen Staniland.
    pages cm
  "Originally published as Volume 35, Issue 2 of The Sociology of Health & Illness"
  Includes bibliographical references and index.
    ISBN 978-1-118-55371-8 (pbk.)
  1. Emerging infectious diseases–Social aspects. 2. World health. 3. Epidemiology. I. Dingwall, Robert, editor of compilation. II. Hoffman, Lily M., editor of compilation. III. Staniland, Karen, editor of compilation. IV. Sociology of Health & Illness.
  RA643.P26 2013
  362.1969–dc23
                        2013017044

A catalogue record for this book is available from the British Library.

Cover design by Design Deluxe.

Set in 9.5/11.5 pt Times NR Monotype by Toppan Best-set Premedia Limited
Printed in Malaysia by Ho Printing (M) Sdn Bhd

1 2013

1

Introduction: why a *sociology* of pandemics?
Robert Dingwall, Lily M. Hoffman and Karen Staniland

This collection explores what sociology has to say about pandemics and emerging infectious diseases at a time when some would claim this topic to be the increasingly exclusive terrain of microbiologists, virologists and practitioners in public health.

Such assertions, we argue, betray a basic lack of understanding of how medicine and biomedical science relate to the world in which they exist. Both are social institutions. This means that they are carried out in social organisations by people who are socially recognised as competent practitioners within a division of labour; that they are delivered through other organisations and through social interactions with innumerable partners. Furthermore, problems come to medicine and biomedical science along socially constructed pathways and are delivered into the world by other pathways: knowledge or technology transfer is a social process. *A focus of attention and resources on medicine and biomedical science, then, tells less than half the story of how societies identify new diseases, how they respond, and what the consequences might be.* In bringing together current work on different aspects of emerging diseases, this monograph also alerts sociological readers to the rich scholarly potential of this area. Emerging diseases are sources of instability, uncertainty and even crises that can make visible features of the social order ordinarily opaque to investigation. As societies respond to these challenges, features that we have taken for granted suddenly become transparent. For a moment, our own world can become anthropologically strange. This is at the core of the contribution made by the sociological imagination to policy and practice, of understanding how social arrangements can, and must, change when biological environments change.

The sociological relevance of new diseases was identified for readers of *Sociology of Health and Illness* by P.M. Strong's (1990) paper on 'Epidemic Psychology'. This title is rather ironic since the paper concerns neither epidemics nor psychology. With the brio for which he was justly celebrated, Strong explored the parallels between what would now be defined as pandemics caused by two emerging infectious diseases: HIV in the 1980s and the Black Death of fourteenth century Europe. Although subsequent research has established that HIV originated in transmission from simian to human populations in West Africa during the early twentieth century (Sharp and Hahn 2011), its emergence and rapid spread across the developing world during the 1980s generated a profound sense of public alarm, particularly in the absence of any effective therapy. This response, Strong argued, resembled that of European populations to the virulent form of bubonic plague that raged across their continent around 1350 (Haensch *et al.* 2010). As institutional memory of an earlier outbreak, Justinian's Plague (541–542 CE), had long been lost, this disease also appeared as a new affliction, with no history, no explanation and no remedy. Both pandemics seemed to threaten the very survival of the societies in which they emerged.

How did these societies react? Although Strong refers to 'social' or 'collective' psychology, his intended audience is sociological: psychology here is used in the sense of Tarde (1901), Park (Elsner, Jr. 1972) or Blumer (1971, McPhail 1989) in their studies of collective behaviour. Strong proposes a sociological study of societal responses to an existential threat. In his own words:

> This essay is a first attempt at a general sociological statement on the striking problems that large, fatal epidemics seem to present to social order; on the waves of fear, panic, stigma, moralising and calls to action that seem to characterise the immediate reaction . . . Societies are caught up in an extraordinary emotional maelstrom which seems, at least for a time, to be beyond anyone's immediate control. Moreover, since this strange state presents such an immediate threat, actual or potential, to public order, it can also powerfully influence the size, timing and shape of the social and political response in many other areas affected by the epidemic (Strong 1990: 249).

Unlike atavistic psychologies which assume that disorder results from primitive emotions unleashed by such threats, Strong argues that apparently bizarre behaviour may be entirely intelligible once it is understood how the world is routinely stabilised by language and social institutions. Emerging diseases disturb our assumptions of a known universe of risk. A new hazard disrupts our established strategies for managing our everyday lives. What appears as irrational may be a locally rational response to uncertainty, or at least an attempt to use locally available resources to re-establish sufficient certainty for practical action.

Underlying Strong's approach is his use of interactionist traditions in US and European sociology – he explicitly pairs Mead and Schutz as his sources of inspiration. These stress the inherent formlessness of the world: it acquires order as the outcome of human actions that assign meaning to events through the socially shared medium of language and the institutions that have evolved to manage and stabilise sources of uncertainty. New diseases are not self-evident and do not direct the societal response. They must be defined by those agents and institutions that are socially licensed to distinguish disease from other kinds of deviance. This definition, in turn, provides a basis for societal mobilisation. Strong focusses on two particularly dramatic cases. At the time he was writing, HIV had only just become stabilised as a result of rapid scientific work that had produced agreement on the identification and nature of the virus in 1986. In the absence of closure by those institutions licensed to declare a matter settled under the impersonal authority of science, rival narratives had competed for authority in much the same way as occurred in the fourteenth century. Was HIV some kind of divine punishment for sin or possibly an evolutionary response to the abuse of human bodies by the consumption of unnatural chemicals or the intensification of non-reproductive sexual practices? The Black Death seemed similarly incomprehensible, particularly as the religious authorities, who were then the main source of closure, were even less well placed than twentieth century scientists to establish a definitive naming and control strategy. In the end, it simply burned out, although outbreaks recurred until the 1750s, and, as Strong remarked in seminar presentations, were accepted as periodic inconveniences that would kill a lot of people but had proved unlikely to bring about the end of humanity.

Thirty years later, however, it has become clear that the shadow cast by HIV, along with subsequent outbreaks of infectious diseases, threats of biological terrorism, and the new vulnerabilities invoked by intense globalisation, prompted a concerted effort to constrain the possibilities for future disorder by what we might call 'stabilisation in advance'. By this we mean the creation of actor-networks that are primed for rapid mobilisation to manage 'known unknowns'. Considerable investments have been made in surveillance, at supra-national, national and subnational levels, to give 'early warnings' of new diseases, to plan for the consequences, and to enhance the resilience of institutions faced with an outbreak. The threat of disorder is never far from the thoughts of those involved – but it is seen as potentially manageable with the resources of a modern society. 'Waves of fear, panic, stigma, moralising and calls to action' are thought to be containable with the application of science, although they may still be invoked in arguments between interested parties.

The collection opens with a group of chapters focussing on the social production of new diseases. By this we mean the processes that turn a disruption of the social ordering of relations between humans and their biological environment into a phenomenon that has been named, classified and assigned a causal account from microbiology or virology. French and Mykhalovskiy discuss the attempts by public health agencies to identify such events as they occur, if not beforehand. Their approach is strongly influenced by Actor-Network Theory (ANT), which also draws inspiration from Tarde's collective psychology (Latour 2002). They characterise public health as an actor-network that creates disease events as the outcome of a joint enterprise that mobilises both human and non-human actants. Emerging diseases are co-constituted by the social and the medical. An emerging infectious disease must marshal and enrol a complex assemblage of scientists, doctors, planners, laws, patients, vectors and the like in order to be recognised: influenza could not fully accomplish this until the 1930s when viruses succeeded in getting themselves distinguished from bacteria, which explains many of the problems encountered in managing both the 1889–90 and 1918–19 influenza pandemics.[1] Gislason approaches the same issues within a Foucauldian framework, which has been widely adopted by the sociology of public health. ANT and Foucauldian analyses take very different positions on the nature of power in society: Latour (1987: 223) declared, 'We need to get rid of all categories like those of power, knowledge, profit or capital, because they divide up a cloth that we want seamless in order to study it as we choose'. In contrast, Gislason sees the constitution of West Nile Virus as an exercise of power by the Public Health Agency of Canada, which articulated a particular reading of the disease, selected a preferred authoritative determination of its nature, and of appropriate interventions, and ultimately normalised it as a routine event in the Canadian biosphere. West Nile Virus is also the focus of Jerolmack's contribution, which examines the problems of establishing ownership of a disease. One characteristic of recent emerging diseases has been their movement from animal to human populations. Animals, or in this case birds, have, however, traditionally been the focus of surveillance systems that work quite independently from those directed at humans, and which tend to concentrate on a limited range of species determined by reference to their economic value. Jerolmack also draws on ANT, to describe the difficult process by which West Nile Virus came to be distinguished within the animal disease reference system and then passed into the human public health system, as a hybrid struggling to reconstitute well-established but segregated organisational networks.

A second group of chapters examine these organisational networks. Chien pursues issues identified by Jerolmack to discuss how international agencies concerned with human health (World Health Organization), agriculture (Food and Agriculture Organization) and animals (World Organization for Animal Health) tried to establish a shared framing of the potential threats from viruses in poultry. These were seen as a likely source for a new influenza pandemic but represented an immediate threat to economically valuable birds. The result was the 'One World, One Health' framework, which was able to serve as a 'boundary object' (Gieryn 1983) that could, at some level, unify the different agencies' efforts, at the cost of a high degree of abstraction and uncertainty in what would constitute implementation. Implementation issues are central to Figuie's case study of Vietnam. The country was seen as a potential epicentre for the emergence of a form of H5N1 influenza capable of easy transmission between humans and, hence, a global pandemic threat. Indeed, virtually the entire international surveillance effort prior to 2009 focussed on South East Asia and South China, assuming that the interactions between human and bird populations in that region were the most likely source of the next pandemic influenza strain. Figuie shows how actions on the ground within Vietnam became entangled with internal political tensions between localism and centralism in government and with an external agenda to complete the country's international rehabilitation following the defeat of the USA in 1975.

Interactions between global and local politics in the management of infectious diseases are further explored by Taylor in comparing responses to HIV by different European states. She notes how Germany, France and the UK manage health threats associated with international migration. All three have a legacy of nineteenth century legislation that empowers them to screen migrants for tuberculosis and to use the results as grounds for quarantine or refusal of entry. However, all three declined to adapt these powers to regulate the movement of people with HIV/AIDS. This, she suggests, reflects the emergence of HIV/AIDS within a context where transnational human rights was a potent discourse, particularly when allied to the project of creating a common European citizenship. This created a collective imaginary within which HIV acquired a different kind of identity from tuberculosis. Such 'disease identities' characterise sufferers in particular ways that endure over time and inform public policies. Hoffman pursues the national/local interplay in a study of New York City's response to H1N1 influenza. Referencing debates within urban sociology about the relative importance of supra-national organisations, nation-states, and global cities, and drawing upon Weber's classic definition of the city as unit of defence, she looks at NYC's response to the 2009 H1N1 outbreak. After 9/11 the reframing of infectious disease as a national security threat under a standardised 'all-hazards' emergency preparedness strategy, contributed to the renewed importance of the city as key actor. When the 'one-size-fits-all' model based on a worst-case scenario failed to provide guidance, the New York Department of Health and Mental Health seized the initiative and imposed its own response strategy. While there may have been important local factors that contributed to the Department's success, Hoffman nevertheless demonstrates that the enactment of public health interventions cannot be simply read off from a national disaster management template: the return of epidemics and the need for defence requires a degree of local autonomy. Also looking at New York City but through the earlier case of West Nile Virus, Whitney and McCormick echo issues identified by French and Mykhalovskiy and by Gislason. Their approach, however, is organisational and institutional, emphasising the impact of emergency powers and the conflict generated by their use, in this case to impose a pesticide spraying regime intended to control the virus's insect vectors. The resulting controversy challenged the legitimacy of the governance regime, with its incentives to adopt this aggressive strategy in preference to more targeted interventions. They note how this questioning led the federal government to respond with intensive investments in attempts to generate legitimacy.

Three chapters look at more detailed aspects of policy implementation. Mansnerus draws on the growing body of sociological work on the rise of quantification as a feature of the contemporary world. She focuses on modelling as a technology for legitimating particular versions of the future as the foundation of current policies and investments. For all their apparent precision, models are essentially a way to black-box a range of issues and uncertainties and produce an authoritative narrative that temporarily stabilises the future. They are a latter-day version of oracles, divination or clairvoyance, deriving their societal licence from science rather than from religion. Steyer and Gilbert investigate the implications of the contemporary movement to frame governance as a collaboration between public authorities and private interests. Their chapter explores the implications of the well-recognised institutional and cultural problems in achieving effective partnerships. Companies struggle with legal and reputational issues, while governments find that they cannot fully delegate responsibilities for public protection. The result is a weak form of co-production that is likely to fail in the crisis it is intended to manage. Godderis and Rossiter take a historical turn to highlight the role of gender in societal responses to pandemic disease. In their short note, they document appeals to women to volunteer as nurses during the 1918 influenza pandemic: their gender placed them under a moral duty to care, regardless of the personal risks or the implications for their families. The nature and limits of the duty to care were particularly exposed during the SARS outbreak in 2002–03, much as they had been during the early years of HIV/AIDS, and became a concern for pandemic response planning (Ruderman *et al.* 2006). Although not fully tested by the relatively mild nature of the 2009 H1N1 influenza pandemic, there was considerable uncertainty about whether social and organisational change might have weakened the force of appeals to this supposed moral duty. How would the conflicting claims of family and profession be resolved by healthcare workers asked to care simultaneously for both and to manage the risks of transmitting infection in either direction?

Finally, three chapters examine public reactions to the 2009 H1N1 pandemic. Staniland and Smith review an international range of studies of media reporting on this pandemic. Although their findings are consistent with Strong's arguments about the initial inflammation of societal anxieties, they show that the difficulty in identifying an unequivocal 'folk devil' quickly diffused these fears. Unlike HIV/AIDS' early identification as a 'gay plague', H1N1 was not easily associated with a consistent cast of villains: it was introduced to the UK via people who had been on expensive package holidays in Mexico. They were not an already stigmatised group who could be further accused of propagating disease. The speed of the issue cycle in news media also meant that representatives of order – scientists, doctors, policymakers – could address and dampen anxieties before panic could set in. Of course, it should be acknowledged that H1N1 proved to be a relatively mild infection and that it was represented as the return of something that science knew about rather than something wholly unfamiliar like HIV. Authority won this framing contest but a similar result may not be guaranteed in the future. This analysis is extended in the short note by Mesch *et al.*, which examines US survey evidence on public responses to media reports. While methodological limitations circumscribe their conclusions, the analysis shows a positive relationship between media consumption and worry, which is accentuated by social status: women, older people and those with larger families became increasingly concerned between May and August 2009. The rise among older people seems particularly worthy of further investigation, given that it emerged over the same period that they were less at risk than children, probably because of some residual cross-immunity from previous influenza pandemics. Sherlaw and Raude show the value of asking counterfactual questions in social science with their inquiry into the absence of panic among the French population. They argue that this was, at least in part, the result of media and policy framing that had anchored future influenza pandemics in the context of the 1918 pandemic. Since 2009 fell so far short of this dramatic possibility, its potential for engendering panic was correspondingly limited. In the absence of popular mobilisation, however, French people showed themselves unwilling to take up vaccination or engage in behavioural measures intended to interrupt the transmission of the virus. There is, Sherlaw and Raude conclude, a fine line between preparedness and alarmism, of generating enough public concern to engage in self-protection and provoking panic. Could the legacy of the perceived exaggeration in invoking the 1918 experience as a template for the 2009 pandemic be a loss of trust in future calls for action by public health agencies? Do they risk the fate of the boy who cried 'wolf' too often?

The chapters in this collection cover a diverse range of countries and diseases. From a sociological perspective, what is striking is the extent to which different emerging diseases provoke common reactions, which are only slightly modified by national environments. Figuie's discussion of central/local tensions in Vietnam is replicated by the studies of New York. Jerolmack's account of the difficulties between the surveillance systems targeted at human and animal diseases is replicated in an as yet unpublished study of Ghana and Malawi.[2] These are not, however, the panicked reactions discussed by Strong or still expected by so many policymakers. Several contributors suggest explanations: the news cycle has accelerated so much that this initial phase of societal reaction flashes past. Public health systems have established better systems of surveillance, early warning and crisis management so that the orderliness of society can be more rapidly re-established. Moreover, the diseases themselves have proved to be containable, susceptible to conventional bioscientific means of analysis and control.

This collection moves beyond the classic sociological focus on societal reactions and the social construction of disease. The reappearance of infectious disease in an intensely globalised arena, marked by supra-national as well as national and local actors, has raised many other issues, including the impact of scientific modalities on uncertainty and risk, the interplay of public health and national security, the dynamics of health governance, and the gendered division of caring labour. It goes without saying that each of these, in turn, raises provocative questions for policy and implementation. In the 21st century, a focus on pandemics and emerging infectious disease gives new insight into evolving social structures and processes. This collection challenges sociologists to contribute further to the public and policy agenda – and questions the narrow thinking that would seek to 'leave it all to biomedical science'.

Acknowledgements

Robert Dingwall has benefitted from numerous discussions with fellow-members of the UK Department of Health Committee on Ethical Aspects of Pandemic Influenza and Roche Pharmaceuticals Pandemic Advisory Council.

Notes

1   This approach was suggested by Gearóid Ó'Cuinn.
2   This draws on discussions with Evanson Sambala.

References

Blumer, H. (1971) Social problems as collective behavior, *Social Problems*, 18, 3, 298–306.
Elsner, Jr., H. (1972) *Robert E Park: The Crowd and the Public and Other Essays*. Chicago: University of Chicago Press.

Gieryn, T.F. (1983) Boundary-work and the demarcation of science from non-science: strains and interests in professional ideologies of scientists, *American Sociological Review*, 48, 6, 781–95.

Haensch, S. et al. (2010) Distinct clones of *yersinia pestis* caused the black death, *PLoS Pathogens*, 6, 10, e1001134. doi:10.1371/journal.ppat.1001134 (accessed 14 October 2012).

Latour, B. (2002) Gabriel Tarde and the end of the social. In Joyce, P. (ed.) *The Social in Question. New Bearings in History and the Social Sciences*. London: Routledge.

Latour, B. (1987) *Science in Action*, Cambridge: Harvard University Press.

McPhail, C. (1989) Blumer's theory of collective behavior: The Development of a Non-Symbolic Interaction Explanation, *The Sociological Quarterly*, 30, 3, 401–23.

Ruderman, C. et al. (2006) On pandemics and the duty to care: whose duty? Who cares? *BMC Medical Ethics*, 7:5 doi:10.1186/1472-6939-7-5 (accessed 14 October 2012).

Sharp, P.M. and Hahn, B.H. (2011) Origins of HIV and the AIDS pandemic, *Cold Spring Harbor Perspectives in Medicine*, 1, 1. Available at: http://www.ncbi.nlm.nih.gov/pmc/articles/PMC32-34451/(accessed 10 September 2012).

Strong, P.M. (1990) Epidemic psychology: a model, *Sociology of Health and Illness*, 12, 3, 249–59.

Tarde, G. (1901) *L'opinion et la foule (1901)*. Paris: Alcan. Available at: http://classiques.uqac.ca/classiques/tarde_gabriel/opinion_et_la_foule/opinion_et_foule.html (accessed 10 September 2012).

2

Public health intelligence and the detection of potential pandemics
Martin French and Eric Mykhalovskiy

Introduction

In what is by far the most commented-upon post on the *Public Health Matters Blog*, Ali S. Khan, Director of the Office of Public Health Preparedness and Response at the United States Centers for Disease Control and Prevention (CDC), instructs readers on how to prepare for a zombie apocalypse – 'That's right, I said z-o-m-b-i-e a-p-o-c-a-l-y-p-s-e' (Kahn 2011). This fanciful piece of health communication hooks readers in with a light-hearted take on the living dead before delivering a more serious message about how to prepare for all kinds of emergencies, ranging from natural disasters to disease pandemics, and even for the zombie apocalypse. If the comparatively huge number of comments on this post are any indication, Kahn's message has resonated with a net-savvy audience.

Beyond disseminating the ideas and discourse of emergency preparedness, Kahn's blog post reflects an emergent effort to cultivate electronic communication about health events. As such, it illustrates a key and novel dimension of contemporary public health intelligence (PHI). A central aim of contemporary PHI is the detection of health events as (or even *before*) they unfold. In the early 20th century, 'epidemiological intelligence' was gathered by health organisations – e.g. regional bodies operating under the auspices of the League of Nations – through a variety of media, including 'wireless broadcast; telegraph; and weekly tabled publications' (Bashford 2006: 73). Today, digitised media have inspired technoscientific imaginaries that render these older media arcane; whereas the intelligence systems of the early 20th century aimed at being 'current' (Lothian 1924), those of the early 21st century are directed ahead of the current. Aspiring towards this pre-emptive ideal means extending PHI beyond traditional activities, such as epidemiological surveillance and the systematic tabulation of case reports, into non-traditional activities such as blogging and data-mining in electronically mediated social networks.

To the extent they get people communicating about the health events they perceive, these non-traditional activities constitute a potential treasure-trove of health-relevant information. Accordingly, Kahn (2011) is engaged not just in cultivating public communication about the zombie apocalypse and other health events, but also in exhorting public health organisations to prepare to mine this treasure-trove for PHI. Capitalising on the 'wisdom of crowds' – leveraging the public's communication about its embodied interactions with

Pandemics and Emerging Infectious Diseases: The Sociological Agenda, First Edition. Edited by Robert Dingwall, Lily M. Hoffman and Karen Staniland. Chapters © 2013 The Authors. Book Compilation © 2013 Foundation for the Sociology of Health & Illness / John Wiley & Sons Ltd.

health-altering exposures – is thought to require significant transformations in public health. New concepts, competencies, forms of knowledge and organisational initiatives are called for – as Kahn *et al.* (2010: 1240) argue:

> Effective fusion of multiple, disparate, and often unstructured and overwhelming streams of data will require the development of new tools and a new cadre of trained public health information analysts, epidemiologists, and informaticians.

It is hoped that such transformations will significantly enhance public health's ability to identify and respond to health events of potential pandemic proportion.

Insofar as they are motivated by pandemic spectres, contemporary developments in PHI – and the associated transformations in public health they initiate – reflect a broader set of time–space relations that are characteristic of contemporary thinking about pandemics. On the one hand, these relations involve a high degree of sensitivity to the spatial dimensions of health events, especially their potential to extend beyond local settings. On the other hand, they are beset by a deep anxiety about the timeliness of response, the outcome of which is an immense effort to detect, pre-empt or rapidly respond to health events to prevent them from having trans-local effects. The matrix of intelligibility set out by these time–space relations calls for particular forms of PHI, and particular ways of organising public health practice.

Our specific interest in this pandemic matrix of intelligibility is with the novel dimensions of PHI it calls into being. These dimensions constitute an important site of empirical investigation for an emergent strand of research within the sociology of public health (SPH). Moreover, their formation in relation to – and imbrication with – spectres of pandemic proportion means that they are interesting for sociological analyses of pandemics. To demonstrate the importance of PHI to the detection and realisation of pandemic phenomena, we first position it as a key, but emergent, focal point within SPH. We then discuss the conceptualisation of pandemics in public health discourse, and their concomitant actualisation in PHI actor-networks. Using the 2009 influenza A (H1N1) pandemic as an example, we consider both the semantic instability of the pandemic concept, and the complex conditions under which pandemics condense 'into specific realities' (van Loon 2005: 40). Finally, using the analytic tools of actor-network theory (ANT) (Latour 2005, Law and Hassard 1999), we suggest some productive – and as yet underdeveloped – sites for empirical research into PHI that can further contribute to the sociology of pandemics.

The sociology of public health (SPH)

In Canada, where we reside, the term 'public health' describes an institution that has population-level health as its focus. This approach – according to the National Advisory Committee on SARS and Public Health (NAC) that assessed the state of Canada's public health system following the 2003 severe acute respiratory syndrome (SARS) epidemic – is based on a recognition 'that the health of populations and individuals is shaped by a wide range of factors in the social, economic, natural, built, and political environments,' all of which may 'interact in complex ways with each other and with innate individual traits such as sex and genetics' (NAC 2003: 19). Given this holistic population-level focus, the work undertaken by public health professionals is frequently rather different from that undertaken by professionals working in clinics or hospitals. As NAC (2003: 2) describes it, public health has several key functions, including:

health protection (e.g., food and water safety, basic sanitation), disease and injury prevention (including vaccinations and outbreak management), population health assessment; disease and risk factor surveillance; and health promotion. [. . .] Public health also plays a key role in disaster and emergency response.

Perhaps owing to its emphasis on populations (as opposed to individuals), the nature of this work can be difficult for citizens to fathom. In NAC's words:

> [the] public health system, unlike the clinical or personal health services system, tends to operate in the background, little known to most Canadians unless there is an unexpected outbreak of disease. (NAC 2003: 19)

Public health's obscure profile, compared with the clinical or personal health services system, is reflected in medical sociology, which has historically accorded greater emphasis to the latter. As an indicator of its somewhat marginal position within the field, major sociological reference texts such as the Oxford *Dictionary of Sociology* or the *Blackwell Encyclopedia of Sociology* devote entries to health care but not to public health. Thus, public health seems to operate in the background not just for citizens, but also for medical sociologists. This is rather surprising given the prominence accorded to public health in other disciplines, such as anthropology (Hahn and Inhorn 2009) or history (Porter 1994).

In spite of its low profile, the SPH constitutes a complex, nuanced, diverse body of work that ranges across several issues and draws on multiple theoretical and methodological traditions. Although it is tempting to divide this work according to whether it is aligned with, or critical of, public health – a division not dissimilar to the one classically identified in medical sociology by Straus (1957) – this would oversimplify the commingling of aligned and critical approaches frequently evident in the SPH. A better way to characterise this work, therefore, is according to its key focal points (Weir and Mykhalovskiy 2010).

An exhaustive review of key focal points in SPH is beyond the scope of this chapter. For present purposes, though, it is worthwhile to consider research on (1) the social determinants of population health; (2) disease prevention, healthy conduct and biological citizenship; as well as (3) PHI.

Social determinants of population health
Sociological engagement with the social determinants of population health has deep roots in research on political economy. In this strand, SPH has directed analytic attention to the relationships amongst capital, the state and civil society whilst harkening back to social justice traditions associated with earlier hygiene movements. Critique is directed at the overemphasis, in public health discourse, on individual, lifestyle health risks. Social, political and economic institutions represent key sites of investigation (Spitler 2001), as does the unequal distribution of economic, social and cultural capital (Raphael 2004). Prescriptions typically call for a transformed public health inclusive of interventions that improve housing, education, employment opportunity, and other structural factors impacting the health of communities and individuals (Coburn *et al.* 2003).

Disease prevention, healthy conduct and biological citizenship
Sociological engagement with disease prevention, healthy conduct and biological citizenship is informed in large measure by Foucaultian analytics. Indebted to Armstrong's (1995) work on 'surveillance medicine' and the concomitant pathologisation of normalcy whereby we are all viewed as 'precariously healthy' and potentially ill (Armstrong 2002: 131), this strand

of SPH directs attention to risk factors and the regulation of lifestyle. Critique focuses on the formation and function of public health expertise, for example, in relation to genetics (Petersen and Bunton 2002), as well as the relationship between health promotion, governance, identity and biological citizenship (Rose 2007). Typically less prescriptive than the social determinants strand, this strand of SPH nonetheless appeals to a democratic ethos by making visible for contestation the subtle forms of contemporary self-governance effected through public health.

Public health intelligence (PHI)
An emergent strand of research, conversant with the above strands of SPH, prioritises the study of PHI – the concepts, methods, practices, and apparatuses assembled to monitor and detect health events (e.g. Donaldson and Wood 2004, Fisher and Monahan 2011, French 2009, Weir and Mykhalovskiy 2010). Events that are recognised to have significance for population health are not simply infectious diseases, but could also include natural disasters, chemical or radiological incidents, explosions, etc. As currently conceptualised within the global regime governing world health, events are distinguished by their potential public health effects. For example, under article 5(3) of the most recent iteration of the International Health Regulations (IHR), the World Health Organization (WHO) is mandated to 'collect information regarding *events* [not just diseases] through its surveillance activities *and assess their potential* to cause international disease spread and possible interference with international traffic' (WHO 2005: 11; added emphasis). Here, the apprehension of health events, and especially their potential to cause trans-local disruption, is key.

Empirical analysis and critique in this strand of SPH has thus far been focused on the 'apparatuses that continuously monitor phenomena that may give rise to catastrophic events' (Weir and Mykhalovskiy 2010: 8), especially as they are articulated by public health professionals. Too nascent to have yet elaborated strongly prescriptive positions, this strand of SPH encourages still more empirical attention to the everyday practices, active concepts, forms of knowledge, diverse informants and organisational initiatives required of PHI apparatuses. As we shall suggest, developments in PHI are driven by – and may recursively amplify – the sense of anxiety evoked by the contemporary conceptualisation of pandemics.

Conceptualisation and actualisation of pandemics

In a recent review of the implementation of the 2005 IHR and the WHO's handling of the 2009 influenza A (H1N1) pandemic, a panel of public health experts concluded that the 'world is ill-prepared to respond to a severe influenza pandemic or to any similarly global, sustained and threatening public-health emergency' (WHO 2011: 12). This sobering conclusion, which stems from the identification of limitations not just in public health capabilities, but also in weak health care delivery systems, the faltering economic development of low- and middle-income countries, and the mediocre health status of many of the world's populations, evokes an epic breadth and depth of impact imagined to inhere in a severe pandemic. Social scientists have picked up on such conceptualisations in contemporary public health discourse – ranging from the preparedness plans of international health organisations to the public statements of local health officials – illustrating their problematic emphasis of uncertainty and the incalculability of pandemic risk (Wraith and Stephenson 2009). Yet little work has thus far been undertaken on PHI efforts to respond to these conceptualisations.

To help explain what is motivating PHI efforts aimed at detecting uncertain and incalculable pandemic risks, we first consider the semantic instability of the pandemic concept. A corollary of this instability is that there are multiple dimensions of pandemic phenomena to which a sociology of pandemics could attend. Nevertheless, as our concern is with PHI, and specifically with the means of actualising pandemics through PHI, we trace the semantic instability surrounding pandemics not solely to struggles over signification, but also to the contingent, often invisible – yet crucial – alliances that condense pandemics into specific realities. In addition to actualising pandemics, these alliances may also broaden the range of phenomena understood in pandemic terms.

Semantic struggles in an enlarged space of pandemic potentiality
Before the 2005 IHR were adopted, the international legal framework governing infectious disease (the 1969 IHR) applied only to traditionally 'quarantinable' conditions, such as cholera (Baker and Fidler 2006: 1058). With the 2005 IHR, the focus shifted from a few listed diseases to the much more broadly conceived notion of *events* that may constitute a public health emergency of international concern. This shift reflects an enlarged conceptual space for thinking about pandemics.

Although a great deal of public health discourse remains preoccupied with the pandemic potential of infectious disease (and, as we are advocating for greater attention to PHI, we share this preoccupation), any number of non-infectious health events could be defined as pandemic in nature – consider recent literature on obesity, for instance (e.g. Swinburn *et al.* 2011). This broad conceptualisation of pandemic potentiality admits multiple possible entry points for a sociology of pandemics. For example, scholarship could attend to the structural inequalities that predispose some populations to higher morbidity and mortality than others as a consequence of pandemic events (Farmer 1999). Or, it could attend to the mass-mediated representation of pandemic events and how the discursive construction of pandemics is implicated in the governance of conduct (Wald 2008). Cognisant of these different ways into a sociology of pandemics, but wishing to take a somewhat different approach, we understand the multiple potential meanings and impacts of pandemics as a key driver of – and as recursively stemming from – developments in PHI.

Because the term 'pandemic' can be applied to such a broad range of phenomena, because the consequences of pandemic events can be so varied, and because there is no definition that admits easy operationalisation, public health professionals and organisations have been challenged to define precisely when health events become pandemic in nature. A clear illustration of this challenge is the controversy surrounding the description and definition of the 2009 H1N1 pandemic (Cohen and Carter 2010). As Doshi (2011: 533) remarks, 'despite ten years of issuing guidelines for pandemic preparedness, [the] WHO has never formulated a formal definition of pandemic influenza'. This inability to proffer a precise definition was linked to wildly different estimates of the impact of H1N1. According to Flahault and Zylberman (2010: 322; notes omitted), 'the WHO announced that there had been 30,000 confirmed cases of H1N1 pandemic influenza, but the same day, the CDC estimated around a million cases'.

To the extent that such discrepancies characterise efforts to define – and produce accurate intelligence about – pandemics, public health professionals have found their assessments subject to challenge. Some went so far as to suggest that the 2009 pandemic was 'fake', and that the WHO's decision to describe influenza A (H1N1) as a pandemic was unduly influenced by vaccine manufacturers (Enserink 2010). In the face of such critique, it is not surprising that public health organisations are keenly interested in the means of achieving more perfect knowledge of pandemic health events.

Settling controversy – allies in the actualisation of pandemics
Studying controversies over exactly how to define and characterise pandemics is a good way to understand not only what is driving developments in PHI, but also how these developments settle (or fail to settle) semantic instability. A long-standing approach to empirical fieldwork in ANT has been to attend to moments of controversy. To settle a controversy, Latour (1987: 31) argues, requires 'bringing friends in', enrolling 'allies' and not just human ones. The more allies one can marshal in support of a statement – such as 'H1N1 was the first influenza pandemic of the 21st century' – the more fact-like it becomes. From an ANT perspective, what is interesting about the H1N1 controversy is the assemblage of actors enrolled to make the pandemic case.

Many actors had to be marshalled – H1N1 itself, of course – but also the diagnosed and their social relations, mediated by rapid modes of international travel. Beyond these actors, still more allies were required: the blood of the diagnosed, for example, and the confirmatory blood-work undertaken by laboratories; the reporting systems that aggregated and tallied suspected and confirmed cases; the 'centers of calculation' (Latour 1987: 215) capable of interpreting and disseminating these data; the bureaucracy governing international flows of information and biomaterial (including local, national, regional and global health organisations, as well as the protocols encoded in the 2005 IHR); a pandemic-planning and response infrastructure (including governments and non-governmental organisations – not least corporations); a global media complex to channel resultant communications about H1N1, etc. The point here is that settling the controversy over the (pandemic) status of H1N1 required much more than the spatio-temporal distribution of H1N1 itself; it also required the support of an extended 'actor-network'.

Latour (2005: 44, 46) uses the term 'actor-network' to indicate that actors are 'never alone in carrying out a course of action', that they are instead always working as part of a 'vast array of entities' that are together more than human. We use actor-networks in this Latourian sense. Applied to the study of PHI, it describes the (sometimes uneasy) alliance of microbes, humans, technoscientific infrastructure and other entities enrolled in the work of mediating a health event. Focusing on actor-networks extends analysis beyond the important, but well-established, social scientific focus on the social construction and hermeneutics of pandemics (e.g. Abeysinghe and White 2011, Blakely 2003), and into the material composition of their actualisation. This approach is useful for illuminating the co-constitution of PHI and pandemics. It directs analytic attention, for example, towards the processes that make pandemic phenomena 'constant' (or not) 'through a series of transformations' (Latour 1999: 58). In other words, it highlights the different nodal points in PHI networks that are both activated by the pandemic orientation of PHI, and that, through their activation, actualise pandemic phenomena.

With ANT in mind, we propose that the apparatuses of PHI involve diverse informants, not just the machinery of surveillance and event detection, but also the establishment of embodied actor-networks capable of sensing and reporting on health events of pandemic potential. Kahn's work (discussed above) is exemplary for the way it addresses these dimensions of PHI. On the one hand, it relates to the technical, and technologically enabled, capabilities of mining networks for health-relevant information that might bring potential pandemics to light. On the other hand, by raising public consciousness about pandemic preparedness and by eliciting the participation of informants in electronically mediated exchanges about pandemic potentiality, it enrols bodies into PHI apparatuses, thereby increasing the scope and sensitivity of pandemic detection. This is not, then, only about mining social networks for health-relevant information; it is also about nurturing and growing them such that they contribute to PHI.

PHI: sites for future research

To sum up the argument thus far, the apparatuses of PHI are an important site of empirical investigation for an emergent strand of research within the SPH. We contend that insofar as these PHI apparatuses are formed in response to – and imbrication with – spectres of pandemic potential, they are also interesting for sociological analyses of pandemics. In order to suggest the promise of this line of research, we delineate below some touchstones for further empirical enquiry. These relate to (1) active concepts; (2) forms of knowledge; (3) diverse informants; and (4) organisational initiatives.

Active concepts
It is possible to identify several 'active concepts' (concepts that provoke legal, political and technical transformations) at work in PHI. We discuss two active concepts below – emerging infectious disease (EID) and situation awareness (SA) – indicating that they are points of critical engagement, but also points of departure for more fulsome ANT-informed analyses of PHI.

The current public health preoccupation with spectres of pandemic proportion has roots in the early 1990s, when the concept of EID began to spread internationally. In tandem with its spread were growing 'demands for surveillance, preparedness, collaboration, and response that operated faster and with more complete information than anything previously imagined' (Weir and Mykhalovskiy 2010: 62). Prior to the internationalisation of the EID concept, established approaches to international communicable disease surveillance had relied largely upon official reporting channels. For example, Fidler (2005) notes that, pre-1995, surveillance relied exclusively on information provided by the governments of WHO member states. Whilst this system gave sovereign states some control over official international flows of information about communicable disease outbreaks occurring in their territories, by the late 20th century it came to be viewed as inadequate. This perceived inadequacy, coupled with heightened perceptions of emergency, prompted public health officials to formalise alternate channels of disease surveillance (Weir and Mykhalovskiy 2010: 106). The internationalisation of EID can thus be said to have increased demand for PHI. It fuelled the creation of an imaginary to which developments in PHI respond, and in which the aim is to detect and even pre-empt health events before they have trans-local effects.

SA is another active concept shaping PHI. It was originally defined in the context of systems engineering as:

> the perception of the elements in the environment within a volume of time and space, the comprehension of their meaning, and the projection of their status in the near future. (Endsley 1995: 36)

In public health, SA has been envisioned as essential in at least three different kinds of settings:

> 1) pre-event/threat situations where a wide range of public health events and threats are assessed, 2) emergency response situation awareness in which detailed assessments of a specific event or threat and public health responses to that threat are monitored, and 3) recovery operations during which the on-going mitigation of preventative efforts to a specific event are monitored. (Rolka *et al.* 2008: 2)

Whilst, as this quotation suggests, the particulars of SA in public health are complex and context dependent, its general form has, in the United States, executive and legislative sanction. As Kahn *et al.* (2010: 1237–8) observe, for example, the concept is referenced in both the Pandemic and All-Hazards Preparedness Act; and Homeland Security Presidential Directive 21. Most noteworthy, for the study of PHI, is the anticipatory nature of SA. The attempt to know the present for the purpose of predicting and controlling the future creates an insatiable requirement for PHI.

Active concepts such as EID and SA mark important points of departure for this analysis because they suggest a preoccupation, in public health discourse, with health events of incalculable pandemic potential. This preoccupation shapes current transformations in public health, orienting it towards phenomena that have not traditionally been core concerns (e.g. radiological events). Such reorientation pushes the limit of what might be considered a public health concern, potentially decentring long-standing epidemiological foci.

Forms of knowledge
The decentring of traditional epidemiological concerns is matched by a parallel shift in the forms of knowledge now being privileged in PHI. At the global level, this shift can be conceptualised in terms of the relation between official and unofficial sources of knowledge. Whilst sociologists have long been concerned to understand the contested place of knowledge – especially lay knowledge (Popay and Williams 1996) – in the production of medical truths, little attention has been paid to the incorporation of unofficial forms of knowledge into PHI apparatuses. This lacuna is surprising, especially since the 2005 IHR (which formally recognise unofficial knowledge such as unverified news reports) have significantly reconfigured the global system of public health knowledge relations (Weir and Mykhalovskiy 2010).

Although a perceived benefit of this reconfiguration is the displacement of sovereign states as the sole knowledge brokers concerning health events in their territories, public health organisations are now having to develop the capacity to investigate unofficial knowledge claims. Some have argued that this reconfiguration produces new international norms concerning the reporting of public health events – less able to cover up outbreaks, states more willingly report them to the WHO. This does not, however, diminish the work demanded of PHI and public health organisations; as reports of health events increase, so too does the work of verifying them (Fearnley 2008).

Diverse informants
One consequence of this incorporation and formalisation of unofficial knowledge has been the ballooning of initiatives experimenting with different kinds of 'infodemiological' techniques and technologies (Eysenbach 2009). The past decade has witnessed the 'unprecedented proliferation' of networked systems capable of collecting, producing and communicating PHI (Castillo-Salgado 2010: 97). Numerous local, national, regional and international organisations – not all of which are within the ambit of the public sector – have organised distributed disease notification networks. An early example was ProMED-mail, established in 1994, and originally created to link electronically the scientist-members of the Program for Monitoring Emerging Diseases (ProMED) (Morse 2007). More recently, countless similar initiatives have emerged. For example:

• In the private sector, Google Flu Trends (http://www.google.org/flutrends) provides a prospective view of influenza search patterns in the United States, whilst the Environmental Systems Research Institute (http://www.esri.com/services/disaster-response/earthquakes/

index.html) is monitoring the geological and social ripple effects of recent earthquakes to provide services for disaster response (Castillo-Salgado 2010).

- Public–private partnerships such as the Global Public Health Intelligence Network (http://www.phac-aspc.gc.ca/gphin/), originally jointly created by the WHO and the Government of Canada, scan electronic media sources for health-relevant information (Mykhalovskiy and Weir 2006).
- Comparable initiatives like HealthMap (http://www.healthmap.org), MediSys (http://medusa.jrc.it), EpiSPIDER (http://www.epispider.org) and BioCaster (http://biocaster.nii.ac.jp) use data from disparate sources to produce global views of communicable disease threats (Brownstein *et al.* 2009).

To the above initiatives could be added efforts to enrol diverse informants – including physicians, nurses, pharmacists, librarians, health news reporters, bloggers, birds, bugs, etc. – into PHI networks. We have already discussed the CDC's *Public Health Matters Blog* as a means of cultivating informants. There are many other means. ProMED-mail, for example, encourages volunteer reporting through its annual Awards for Excellence in Outbreak Reporting on the Internet. In 2005, it awarded an anonymous rapporteur for work done to uncover avian influenza reports. That this award was given anonymously is indicative of the risks of reprisal that individual informants can face when they disclose information about health events that sovereign states might wish to keep secret.

In addition to human informants, it is important also to consider non-human informants in the production of PHI. In Canada, efforts to produce knowledge about West Nile Virus (WNV) suggest how non-humans can be enrolled into PHI actor-networks. WNV is an arborovirus that can cause diseases such as meningitis and encephalitis. According to the Public Health Agency of Canada (PHAC), it is spread by mosquitoes that have fed on the blood of infected birds. The virus has been identified in many bird species in North America, and some birds, such as crows and blue jays, become ill and can die from infection with WNV (PHAC 2009). Accordingly, initiatives to track WNV have involved wildlife disease surveillance, including the collection and testing of dead birds and mosquitoes for the presence of the virus (Canadian Cooperative Wildlife Health Centre (CCWHC) 2012). In this example, the embodied exposure of birds and mosquitoes to WNV is enrolled in a broader network of actors to produce PHI. Public health authorities rely on the public to collect and submit birds and mosquitoes for testing. This provides a means of gauging the presence of WNV in a territory before it manifests symptomatically in humans.

Organisational initiatives
To parse information produced by early warning initiatives effectively, public health organisations have been experimenting with ways of becoming more informatically competent. Truly leveraging such early-warning actor-networks for PHI is thought to require major shifts in organisational culture. As Kahn *et al.* (2010: 1237) argue, nothing less than 'an information revolution' is required. Looking to the post-9/11 intelligence community, which is viewed as having fostered 'a culture of sharing information' (Kahn *et al.* 2010: 1238; note omitted), they identify the development of *fusion centres* as potentially useful to public health, in that they may enhance the collection, analysis, exchange and interpretation of information 'from existing traditional systems and nontraditional sources' (Kahn *et al.* 2010: 1238). Fusion centres are organisations dedicated to bringing together information from distributed sources for manifold purposes. According to the Electronic Privacy Information Center (EPIC), an American public interest research group, the idea for such

organisations originated in the US Department of Defense (DOD). In 2002, EPIC (2012) reports, 'the *New York Times* disclosed a massive DOD fusion center project [. . .] known as Total Information Awareness (TIA) [. . . and meant] to detect terrorists through analyzing troves of information'.

Not mentioning the political controversy surrounding TIA, Kahn *et al.* (2010) describe a CDC fusion centre pilot programme called BioPHusion. Meant to test the operational capacity of public health fusion centres, BioPHusion aimed to enhance agency-wide SA by aggregating, analysing and sharing data from multiple sources across programme areas (Gerberding, cited in Rolka *et al.* 2008: 3). Among other elements, BioPHusion required the acquisition of information sources. It made use of publicly available information such as news media reports; however, as Rolka *et al.* (2008: 4) indicate, its future success would hinge upon the integration of sources from 'environmental monitoring systems, animal or vector monitoring systems, individuals, laboratories, medical records, administrative records, police records, and vital records'.

Such novelties as we have discussed represent only the smallest tip of the iceberg. A great deal of mapping remains to be done, especially as new active concepts, forms of knowledge, informants and organisational initiatives emerge.

Conclusion

We have argued that public health intelligence (PHI) has changed in some significant ways, involving activities that extend beyond the traditional remit of public health. To gesture towards the larger implications of these changes for public health – and for the diverse publics it serves – we would like to underscore two points.

First, to the extent that developments in contemporary PHI have been discussed in the scholarly literature, the concentration has been largely upon the miracle of technology (Morse 2007). Accordingly, the three strands of SPH that we have identified stand to offer new insight into how PHI actually works, and on its larger implications. For instance, little sustained attention has been devoted to the way that PHI actor-networks function in practice. Key questions regarding, for example, the way that public health professionals and other informants enter into these networks remain unanswered. Another set of questions relates to how PHI will be used over the long-term. The development of fusion centres in public health may indicate a growing synergy between the apparatuses of PHI and those of national security intelligence. Such synergy has implications for the institution of public health, specifically whether or not it is set up to serve the comparatively narrow interests of national security or the broader interests of global population health. In addition, key questions remain to be addressed with respect to: (1) whether PHI will lead to improvements in housing, education, employment opportunity and other structural determinants of health; and (2) how PHI will be implicated in the governance of healthy conduct.

A second point to underscore is that the imbrication of PHI with spectres of pandemic potential may be generative of public health institutions – and publics – that are increasingly oriented by pandemic anxiety. Such conditions seem to require 'anticipatory measures to have been systematically put in place across the entire society in order to anticipate the potentially unlimited class of what *might* happen' (Heyman *et al.* 2010: 214; original emphasis). According to our ANT-informed analysis, a key anticipatory measure is the enrolling of diverse informants into PHI actor-networks. This process indicates a reconceptualisation of informants and the publics they constitute. In effect, what we may be witnessing is not simply the enrolment of diverse publics into PHI, but also the constitution of these very publics – especially their networked, embodied interactions with health-altering exposures – *as anticipatory measures*.

To conclude, it is not every day that populations are alerted to a pandemic emergency such as the zombie apocalypse. Whilst the novelty of this alert is noteworthy for the impressive public response it garnered, its greater significance arguably lies in the way it potentially enrols diverse informants into PHI. Indeed, insofar as people communicate their perceptions of the public's health, these are made available for PHI. The CDC's *Public Health Matters Blog* may thus be regarded as much more than an effort to raise public awareness about health events; it is also an effort to create and cultivate networks, which can then be mined for health-relevant information.

In this chapter we have suggested that a sociology of pandemics would benefit from the study of PHI. We have situated the study of PHI as an emergent strand of research within the sociology of public health (SPH). We have also indicated, by focusing on the actor-networks that actualise pandemics (that condense them into specific realities), the broad range of actors involved in bringing health events of pandemic potential to light. Insofar as PHI actor-networks are formed in relation to – and imbrication with – pandemic potentiality, they represent an interesting site of study for the sociology of pandemics. To showcase sites for further research in this vein of enquiry, we briefly discussed key active concepts, forms of knowledge, diverse informants and organisational forms of contemporary PHI. The rise to prominence of these elements in the PHI apparatus indicates not simply a transformation of the institution of public health, but also a reconceptualisation of the *publics* served by this institution.

Acknowledgements

No text comes to light without the affordances of an extended network of interlocutors and friends, and the authors would like to thank theirs for helping them to bring this text to light. In addition, Martin French thanks the Social Sciences and Humanities Research Council of Canada for supporting his research through a Postdoctoral Fellowship. Eric Mykhalovskiy thanks the Canadian Institutes of Health Research for supporting his research through a New Investigator Award.

References

Abeysinghe, S. and White, K. (2011) The avian influenza pandemic: discourses of risk, contagion and preparation in Australia, *Health Risk and Society*, 13, 4, 311–26.

Armstrong, D. (1995) The rise of surveillance medicine, *Sociology of Health & Illness*, 17, 3, 393–404.

Armstrong, D. (2002) A New History of Identity: A Sociology of Medical Knowledge. Houndmills: Palgrave.

Baker, M. and Fidler, D. (2006) Global public health surveillance under new International Health Regulations, *Emerging Infectious Disease*, 12, 7, 1058–65.

Bashford, A. (2006) Global biopolitics and the history of world health, *History of the Human Sciences*, 19, 1, 67–88.

Blakely, D. (2003) Social construction of three influenza pandemics in the New York Times, *Journalism and Mass Communication Quarterly*, 80, 4, 884–902.

Brownstein, J., Freifeld, C. and Madoff, L. (2009) Digital disease detection – harnessing the web for public health surveillance, *New England Journal of Medicine*, 360, 21, 153–7.

Canadian Cooperative Wildlife Health Centre (CCWHC) (2012) *West Nile Virus.* Saskatoon, SK: CCWHC. http://www.ccwhc.ca/west_nile_virus.php (accessed 29 April 2012).

Castillo-Salgado, C. (2010) Trends and directions of global public health surveillance, *Epidemiologic Reviews*, 32, 1, 93–109.

Coburn, D., Denny, K., Mykhalovskiy, E., McDonough, P., Robertson, A. and Love, R. (2003) Population health in Canada: a brief critique, *American Journal of Public Health*, 93, 3, 392–6.

Cohen, D. and Carter, P. (2010) WHO and the pandemic flu 'conspiracies', *British Medical Journal*, 340, 7759, 1274–9.

Donaldson, A. and Wood, D. (2004) Surveilling strange materialities: categorisation in the evolving geographies of FMD biosecurity, *Environment and Planning D*, 22, 3, 373–91.

Doshi, P. (2011) The elusive definition of pandemic influenza, *Bulletin of the World Health Organization*, 89, 7, 523–38.

Electronic Privacy Information Center (EPIC) (2012) *Information Fusion Centers and Privacy.* Washington, DC: EPIC. http://epic.org/privacy/fusion/ (accessed 1 December 2012).

Endsley, M. (1995) Toward a theory of situation awareness in dynamic systems, *Human Factors*, 37, 1, 32–64.

Enserink, M. (2010) Facing inquiry, WHO strikes back at 'fake pandemic' swine flu criticism, Science Insider, 14 January. http://www.news.sciencemag.org/scienceinsider/2010/01/facing-inquiry.html (accessed 27 July 2011).

Eysenbach, G. (2009) Infodemiology and infoveillance: framework for an emerging set of public health informatics methods to analyze search, communication and publication behaviour on the internet, *Journal of Medical Internet Research*, 11, 1, http://www.jmir.org/2009/1/e11/ (accessed 1 December 2012).

Farmer, P. (1999) *Infections and Inequalities: The Modern Plagues.* Berkeley, CA: University of California Press.

Fearnley, L. (2008) Signals come and go: syndromic surveillance and styles of biosecurity, *Environment and Planning A*, 40, 7, 1615–32.

Fidler, D. (2005) From international sanitary conventions to global health security: the new International Health Regulations, *Chinese Journal of International Law*, 4, 2, 1–68.

Fisher, J. and Monahan, T. (2011) The 'biosecuritization' of healthcare delivery: examples of post- 9/11 technological imperatives, *Social Science and Medicine*, 72, 4, 545–52.

Flahault, A. and Zylberman, P. (2010) Influenza pandemics: past, present and future challenges, *Public Health Reviews*, 32, 1, 319–40.

French, M. (2009) Woven of war-time fabrics: the globalization of public health surveillance, *Surveillance and Society*, 6, 2, 101–15.

Hahn, R. and Inhorn, M. (eds) (2009) *Anthropology and Public Health: Bridging Differences in Culture and Society*, 2nd edition. Oxford: Oxford University Press.

Heyman, B., Shaw, M., Alaszewski, A. and Titterton, M. (2010) *Risk, Safety, and Clinical Practice: Health Care Through the Lens of Risk.* Oxford: Oxford University Press.

Kahn, A. (2011) *Preparedness 101: zombie apocalypse, Public Health Matters Blog.* Atlanta, GA: Centres for Disease Control and Prevention (CDC). http://blogs.cdc.gov/publichealthmatters/2011/05/preparedness-101-zombie-apocalypse/ (accessed 27 July 2011).

Kahn, A., Fleischauer, A., Casani, J. and Groseclose, S. (2010) The next public health revolution: public health information fusion and social networks, *American Journal of Public Health*, 100, 7, 1237–42.

Latour, B. (1987) *Science in Action: How to Follow Scientists and Engineers Through Society.* Cambridge, MA: Harvard University Press.

Latour, B. (1999) *Pandora's Hope: Essays on the Reality of Science Studies.* Cambridge, MA: Harvard University Press.

Latour, B. (2005) *Reassembling the Social: An Introduction to Actor-Network-Theory.* Oxford: Oxford University Press.

Law, J. and Hassard, J. (eds) (1999) *Actor Network Theory and After.* Oxford: Blackwell.

Lothian, N. (1924) The service of epidemiological intelligence and public health statistics, *American Journal of Public Health*, 14, 4, 287–90.

Morse, S. (2007) Global infectious disease surveillance and health intelligence, *Health Affairs*, 26, 4, 1069–77.

National Advisory Committee on SARS and Public Health (NAC) (2003) Learning from SARS: Renewal of Public Health in Canada. Ottawa, ON: Health Canada.

Mykhalovskiy, E. and Weir, L. (2006) The Global Public Health Intelligence Network and early warning outbreak detection: a Canadian contribution to global public health, *Canadian Journal of Public Health*, 97, 1, 42–4.

Petersen, A. and Bunton, R. (2002) *The New Genetics and the Public's Health*. London: Routledge.

Popay, J. and Williams, G. (1996) Public health research and lay knowledge, *Social Science and Medicine*, 42, 5, 759–68.

Porter, D. (ed.) (1994) *The History of Public Health and the Modern State*. Amsterdam: Rodopi.

Public Health Agency of Canada (PHAC) (2009) *West Nile Virus: Surveillance, Education, Prevention and Response*. Ottawa, ON: PHAC. http://www.phac-aspc.gc.ca/wn-no/surveillance-eng.php (accessed 29 April 2012).

Raphael, D. (2004) *Social Determinants of Health: Canadian Perspectives*. Toronto, ON: Canadian Scholars' Press.

Rolka, H., O'Connor, J. and Walker, D. (2008) Public health information fusion for situation awareness. in Zeng, D., Chen, H., Rolka, H. and Lober, W. (eds) *Biosurveillance and Biosecurity: Lecture Notes in Computer Science*. Berlin: Springer.

Rose, N. (2007) *The Politics of Life Itself: Biomedicine, Power, and Subjectivity in the Twenty-First Century*. Princeton, NJ: Princeton University Press.

Spitler, H. (2001) Medical sociology and public health: problems and prospects for collaboration in the new millennium, *Sociological Spectrum*, 21, 3, 247–63.

Straus, R. (1957) The nature and status of medical sociology, *American Sociological Review*, 22, 2, 200–04.

Swinburn, B., Sacks, G., Hall, K., McPherson, K., Finegood, D., Moodie, M. and Gortmaker, S. (2011) The global obesity pandemic: shaped by global drivers and local environments, *Lancet*, 378, 9793, 804–14.

Van Loon, J. (2005) Epidemic space, *Critical Public Health*, 15, 1, 39–52.

Wald, P. (2008) *Contagious: Cultures, Carriers, and the Outbreak Narrative*. Durham, NC: Duke University Press.

Weir, L. and Mykhalovskiy, E. (2010) *Global Public Health Vigilance: Creating a World on Alert*. New York, NY: Routledge.

World Health Organization (WHO) (2005) *International Health Regulations*, 2nd edn. Geneva: WHO.

World Health Organization (WHO) (2011) *Implementation of the International Health Regulations (2005): Report of the Review Committee on the Functioning of the International Health Regulations (2005) in Relation to Pandemic (H1N1) 2009*. Geneva: WHO.

Wraith, C. and Stephenson, N. (2009) Risk, insurance, preparedness and the disappearance of the population: the case of pandemic influenza, *Health Sociology Review*, 18, 3, 220–33.

3

West Nile virus: The production of a public health pandemic

Maya K. Gislason

The proliferation of disciplinary institutions and regimes of regulatory controls designed to govern health risks is concurrent with newly emerging and re-emerging infectious disease (EID) pandemics. Reflecting present-day preoccupations with pandemic threats, and faced with complex and novel interactions between microbes, hosts, vectors and environments, the World Health Organization (WHO) has framed the contemporary moment through a prism of pandemics, with moments of reprieve defined as 'inter-pandemic periods' (WHO 2005: vi). Infectious diseases research in medical sociology is beginning to take note (Tausig *et al.* 2006, Timmermans and Haas 2008, Washer 2010) and is offering critiques of the proliferation of disciplinary apparatuses in public health (Petersen and Lupton 1997, Senellart 2007, Mukherjea 2010). Critical perspectives informing this work range from social constructionist studies of EIDs showing that, in the age of modernity and globalisation, emergence events are entwined with politics, economics and governance issues (Petersen and Bunton 1997, Price-Smith 2001). Biomedical and epidemiological research is showing how disease emergences can be products of novel interrelationships between microbes, hosts, vectors and environments that are in turn shaped by forces of globalisation (Gonzales *et al.* 2010, McMichael and Butler 2007, Waltner-Toews 2007). The phenomenon of emergence (see also Stephenson and Jamieson 2009), and in particular that of newly emerging diseases, is an exquisite exemplar of how infectious diseases generate socio-medical responses that are driven not only by concerns that humans can be affected and but also by the perceived threat that they will increase in incidence and spread across national boundaries.

This chapter focuses on the Public Health Agency of Canada's (PHAC) response to the West Nile virus (WNV) epidemic that emerged in Canada in 2004 and shows how PHAC's efforts to promote the health of Canadians not only produced, but were also produced by, specific social relations of power. Studying the emergence of the WNV pandemic within a grid of relations shows that a variety of forces, including biomedical responses, public health governance frameworks and collective social behaviour, contoured the development of PHAC's response to the WNV. PHAC did not simply offer public health guidance but also generated institutional mandates, technological innovations and social responses to patterns of fear and cultural expectations about health. New physical spaces were also designed and built to house governmental administrative developments and regulatory decision-making bodies, public health administrative elaborations, as well as further scientific research

Pandemics and Emerging Infectious Diseases: The Sociological Agenda, First Edition. Edited by Robert Dingwall, Lily M. Hoffman and Karen Staniland. Chapters © 2013 The Authors. Book Compilation © 2013 Foundation for the Sociology of Health & Illness / John Wiley & Sons Ltd.

initiatives. Overall, PHAC's response was not only about a zoonotic disease but also the product of a melange of concrete acts and specific forms of knowledge, making this disease event an effect of power.

Foucauldian theories of power

In medical sociology Foucauldian theories of power have influenced how scholars think about the production of disease (Turner 1997). Foucauldian theories understand power as a cluster of relations as well as a whole set of instruments, techniques, and procedures (Foucault 1995: 215). In this study I have used the notion of a grid – the relationships, structures and effects – to observe how power has been produced and circulated through PHAC's WNV response (Foucault 1980a: 199). Three concepts have been particularly useful. The first is discourse and how power operates in the social world through texts and their materialisation as 'social practices and specific activities that sustain and reproduce discursive formations' (Moss and Dyck 2002: 15). A discourse can reformulate a body of heterogeneous ideas from diverse sources into a single collection of texts but can also embody sets of ideas in 'technical processes, in institutions, in patterns for general behaviour, in forms for transmission and diffusion, and in pedagogical forms which, at once, impose and maintain them' (Foucault 1973: 200). On the PHAC website discourses were central to the construction of the WNV as a health threat because they were productive, dynamic and catalytic, ultimately triggering the production of other discourses and new social realities in relation to the perceived dangers of the WNV. Accordingly, during the emergence of the WNV in Canada, discourses on the PHAC website were at once a medium through which PHAC produced ideas about the WNV and simultaneously a mechanism that reveals the construction process (Foucault 1980b: 101).

The second concept, power/knowledge, highlights the interconnectedness between practices of power and the production of knowledge and how, after becoming intelligible to the social world through the acquisition of form, knowledge assumes authority as a social entity. Power/knowledge is useful for thinking about the construction of the parameters of possibility of PHAC's responses to WNV (Rouse 1994: 95). These occurred within the framework of modern governmentality, within the social and biomedical assumption that knowledge produced through scientific positivism is authoritative. The political milieu was that of a risk culture where notions of fear, threat, and disharmony circulated widely, ultimately linking pandemic emergence to perceptions of global health insecurity caused by microbial activity.

Finally, and perhaps most influential for this study, is the nuanced distinction between technologies and techniques of power. The exercise of power is a technology that assembles various techniques into a single machinery (Foucault 1980b: 140). Technologies operate on the scale of institutions and governments by combining various elements of social and economic reality, according to specific sets of rules and with the purpose of controlling populations (Ewald 1991: 197). Techniques of power are more subtle, as they are the mechanisms, procedures, tools, and skills that turn discipline into the art of delicate and detailed transformations. Though there are multiple techniques through which power as a technology is enacted, and while each technique of power functions in a unique way, when they work together these mechanisms form 'a closely linked grid of disciplinary coercions whose purpose is in fact to assure the cohesion of the social body' (Foucault 1980a: 106). One use for these techniques of power is to craft a public health regime that protects populations in the face of a pandemic threat.

Foucault often uses biomedical and social responses to epidemics as a way to illustrate the production of disciplinary apparatuses (Foucault 2003, Senellart 2007) with attention to place and time as a further method for highlighting the modern dimensions of the phenomenon of disease in society. Foucault observes, for example, that in modern societies diseases are framed as infiltrators on the basis that by their 'birthright, forms and seasons they are alien to the space of society' (2003: 17). A savage character is also given to diseases: a subject on which post-Foucauldian sociologists of risk and governmentality have fruitfully expanded (Beck 1992, 1995, Petersen 1997). The WNV was also denatured on the website, an occurrence linked not only to medicalisation (Conrad 1992, Laing 1964) but also to the complexification of society (Foucault, 2003: 17–18; see also Armstrong 1997, Conrad 1995, Martin 1994, Shilling 2005). Foucault's insights into the roles played by social expectations, identities and relations of power in producing perceptions of health, illness and disease were also useful for reading the PHAC website as an interweaving of ideas and practices (Bendelow et al. 2002, Birke 2002, Busfield 2002, Moss and Dyck 2002). Finally, Foucault was acutely aware of issues of inequity and risk in relation to disease – also evidenced in my own research in public health (Gislason 2010).

Methodology

In this social constructionist, Foucauldian discourse analysis, I approached the WNV not as a biological viral entity but as a conceptual assemblage produced through social relations of power. The PHAC website provided the textual data, as it is an authoritative resource on the WNV in Canada and the product of a number of activities performed by PHAC personnel and other experts – scientists, medical practitioners, public health officials and governmental administrators. This virtual space has played a central role in framing the WNV as a public health issue, distributing authoritative information about the disease, informing citizens about how they can best protect themselves against the threat, and, perhaps ironically, raising anxiety about its epidemic dimensions. In total, 49 webpages were analysed using NVivo. The PHAC's WNV homepage served as the first document and the subsequent 48 texts were those constituting the nine sub-directories: (i) symptoms, (ii) general information, (iii) protect yourself and your family, (iv) First Nations, (v) animals, (vi) surveillance, (vii) maps and statistics, (viii) public education resources and (ix) links.

The analytic method was inspired by Jennifer Gore's identification of eight technologies of power described by Foucault in his work on disciplinary societies: surveillance, normalisation, exclusion, classification, distribution, individualisation, totalisation and regulation (Gore 1997: 2; see also Gore 1995, 2002). In this study, I have elaborated on these analytical categories by adding an analytical layer of micro-techniques. Table 1 illustrates this with examples from four of the eight categories: surveillance, normalisation, exclusion and regulation.

The following analysis of these categories illustrates how relations of power worked together in specific places, spaces and moments in time to construct an identifiable set of (often subtle) ideas about, and practices surrounding, the emergence of the WNV disease.

PHAC's production of the WNV

This section presents four (surveillance, normalisation, exclusion and regulation) of the eight analyses conducted using Foucauldian concepts of power. Significantly, while each

Table 1 *Operationalising Foucault: examples of four technologies of power and their micro-techniques*

	Classic surveillance	*Explicit, hierarchical, state-operated forms of control*
Surveillance	Surveillance through knowledge	Knowledge produced through classical surveillance techniques used to describe how people should discipline themselves and others
	Relations of surveillance	Detected over time in shifts in discourses about appropriate attitudes and behaviour for people to adopt
Normalisation	Defining the field of normalcy	The techniques, people and resources cited in descriptions of what falls inside and outside of the realm of normal thoughts, ideas, and practices
	Content of normalcy	The types of knowledge, practices, and relations that were defined as normal
	Reproduction of normalcy	The methods used to replicate social norms and to ensure that the discourses would not challenge current conventions or lead people lacking the social authority to reshape control and prevention practices or to reconceptualise or elaborate upon the officially sanctioned protocols
Exclusion	Conceptual exclusion	The exclusion of specific ideas, concepts, and words
	Physical exclusion	The marginalisation or exclusion of specific bodies or groups of bodies – an effect accomplished by denaturalising or defining certain bodies as threatening and as requiring removal from specific spaces or places
	Geographical exclusion	The practice of excluding from the social sphere particular spaces, places, and environments were excluded on the basis that they were pathological
Regulation	Subjects of regulation	The people, subjects, activities and forms of knowledge and practice being formally regulated
	Formality of regulation	The scale, kind, formality and force of specific regulations and regulatory practices applied to social actors
	Rationale for regulation	The power/knowledge relations at work in a particular governance situation
	Apparatuses of regulation	Organisations, individuals and groups involved in specific regulatory processes, often linked through a grid of regulatory functions

strategy of power produces its own set of effects, this analysis also shows how, when they are read together, the public health sector can produce a disease to be something other than a biological category and how a public health response can be driven by social forces and not only by considerations about the microbiological, environmental and biomedical dimensions of an EID.

Surveillance
The PHAC plays an important role within Canada's health and security planning. This made it central to framing and reframing the WNV as a significant and widespread health

risk (PHAC 2004). Surveillance, a technique that makes entities visible in order to study, regulate, protect and control them, plays a pivotal role in constructing knowledge about the dangers of EIDs like the WNV and producing a public health response. A social constructionist analysis, however, offers some novel insights. PHAC made the WNV visible through techniques of observation that tracked the activities of the people, animals, insects and environments implicated in the transmission and survival of the WNV in North America with a focus on its activities in Canada that soon brought it from an emergence to a pandemic status. Surveillance linked the, now observable, bodies implicated in the WNV outbreaks and the places being scrutinised to a range of disciplinary practices by PHAC and its partners. Surveillance occurred at four scales and their corresponding arenas. The first arena was the nation-state. Here, the entire population, and the geographical expanses within Canada's borders, were placed under observation. To do this, PHAC analysed and displayed spatial data using technologies such as satellites and geographical information systems. Scientists who study patterns of disease development were among those using these technologies, mapping tools and modelling techniques to produce real-time and predictive epidemiological maps of the WNV outbreaks in Canada. After the nation-state, the second arena of surveillance was the region, in which the province, municipality, reserve and neighbourhood were put under surveillance. Technologies used in regional surveillance programmes included scientists trained in infectious disease surveillance, all-terrain vehicles, digital cameras and hand-held devices programmed to record data about the WNV infection. The third arena was that of the individual. Here, PHAC conducted active surveillance on groups through observation and also relied on groups to observe themselves. Scientists and governmental authorities as well as individuals, who turned the disciplinary gaze both onto themselves (self-surveillance) and onto one another (intersubjective surveillance), are the people who conduct surveillance in this arena. Finally, the fourth arena was that of the organism. Surveillance here requires microscopic technology capable of seeing what is happening inside biological bodies. Laboratory technicians conducted front-line testing using a microscope to scrutinise blood samples from humans and birds for markers of the presence of the WNV. When blood assays do not conclusively locate a WNV virus, physicians conduct confirmatory testing by cross-referencing epidemiological data with laboratory data to confirm that the WNV has been active in the geographical area in which a person had been provisionally diagnosed. Medical practitioners in the clinic, hospital room or operating theatre, as well as scientists in laboratory settings, were among those conducting surveillance at the level of the organism.

On the PHAC website the technique of surveillance produces specific knowledge about the WNV and its threats, which was used instrumentally within a variety of formal responses to the disease. As the website explains:

> Human surveillance information is used in a number of important ways. Knowing that West Nile virus is in an area puts doctors and the general public on alert. It also provides more clues about who may be at risk for serious health effects from West Nile virus. In addition, human surveillance provides information to help ensure the safety of the blood supply in Canada. (PHAC 2004b)

Each way that surveillance is utilised points to a relation of power at work within PHAC's production of the WNV. As the passage above indicates, PHAC conducts surveillance to locate the position of WNV activity spatially, as well as to gather data that can be used to contextualise the WNV socially. For instance, on the PHAC website the word 'alert' highlights the notion that the WNV is a viral invader that has breached the Canadian border while the words 'area' and 'risk' convey the message that the WNV is an active health threat in communities and neighbourhoods. By distributing the message that the WNV is a threat in our midst, PHAC raises the public's level of awareness about the WNV and, because this message is presented as an alert, it may also lead people who live in the areas under surveillance and/or who feel personally vulnerable to WNV infection to feel a heightened awareness of the presence of the WNV. To reinforce the idea that people should personalise the threat from the WNV, PHAC uses the pronoun 'who' to indicate to whom it is directing particular messages about the threat. Correspondingly, PHAC places these same people under observation or delegates to them the task of observation. PHAC's prevention literature, for instance, suggests that individuals, especially those deemed to be more at risk of becoming ill from a WNV infection (such as older adults and pregnant women), watch their behaviour and health closely (PHAC 2012). Finally, PHAC's reference to the blood supply underscores the biological dimensions of the WNV and, in doing so, offers another rationale, albeit indirect in this framing, for PHAC's use of the scientific method to produce knowledge about, and responses to, the WNV.

Analysing the PHAC website through surveillance as a technique of power illustrates that PHAC relies upon observation in various arenas to make the WNV visible. Once visible, PHAC can use the WNV to rationalise the agency's investment in surveillance as a preventive health strategy and to justify the proliferation of new surveillance technologies, the allocation of more federal funds, the assignment of certain places and groups under surveillance and the use of surveillance data to generate knowledge about the WNV. Through spatial demarcations of the presence of the WNV, PHAC is able to produce the WNV as something other than just a biological entity, namely, as a health threat that needs close ongoing scrutiny. In sum, through surveillance PHAC establishes the scope, and demarcates the terrain, of its WNV responsibilities and reach, including the spaces it will oversee, the people it will track (in an effort to protect them) and the animals and insects that are factors in its programme.

Normalisation
The entire PHAC website is a technique of normalisation. Normalisation is more than the governing of people's actions through norms (read: socialisation): it is a technique through which norms order and shape all aspects of social life. As a technique of power, normalisation is used on the PHAC's website to define and regulate what is appropriate, customary, routine, regular, familiar, acceptable and expected (PHAC 2009). However, as the concept of normality changes over time, judges of normality must participate in the production and reproduction of normality by subjecting individual gestures, behaviour, comportment and aptitudes to repeated scrutiny. PHAC has produced its website to function in much the same way as a judge of normality, to define appropriate prevention activities and to invoke the WNV infection as the ultimate consequence of failing to comply with its prevention plans. By combining individualisation with normalisation (see Foucault 1973, 1980b, 1995 and 2003), PHAC produces the message that responsible individuals monitor their own behaviour, as well as the actions of others, and that failure to do this will lead to illness, if not death. In addition, the material on the website serves to normalise PHAC's construction of the WNV and its response to this new infectious disease pandemic by suggesting that what it is doing and saying as Canada's public health agency is socially responsible, scientifically reliable and politically sound (Health Canada 2006). PHAC produces this effect in part by invoking the authority of the scientific method, which it equates with scientific positivism or the ability to produce objective, factual knowledge about social and biological

phenomena. PHAC's authoritative approach is also normalised because of the agency's political location and access to economic resources to reproduce its approach and to widely distribute the material it generates.

PHAC also capitalises on its authority and affiliation to scientific expertise to justify the exclusion of contradictory viewpoints: for example, by using quotes from governmental officials and scientists who define what is normal and acceptable and, by extension, what is abnormal and unacceptable about the WNV and the responses it demands of the public health sector. The nine main sections on PHAC's WNV website were elsewhere reformatted as fact sheets designed to be downloaded and distributed. The underlying assumptions normalised in these fact sheets include the idea that the expectations placed on the public in the health promotion and campaign literature are acceptable and the activities the public is asked to engage in are rooted in the most salient common sense and scientific knowledge. In staking the territory of presenting 'facts' PHAC also undermines the authority of others, especially reactions from groups or individuals that challenge the programme. Drawing attention to the language and techniques of normalisation also allows for the identification of the role of positivist science in the production of authoritative knowledge and raises questions about the absence of complexity science or information about the interaction between microbial activities and various socio-ecological contexts of emergence. In other words, the predominately simplified messages presented on the website miss an opportunity to engage with the complexity of the WNV presence in Canada.

By extension, this approach to presenting health information to the public allows the PHAC website to act as a strong normalising force in defining the WNV and setting up the parameters for appropriate responses to this newly emergent infectious disease. These parameters, in part due to the authority PHAC holds in the arena of public health, are reproduced in society and, consequently, inform a variety of less formal institutional and individual responses to the WNV. Readers of the website are expected to become advocates for rejecting alternative (read. unscientific and therefore unreliable) views. The normalisation process that is already produced through PHAC's WNV website is therefore reinforced by the concerned reader.

Exclusion

Another way that effects of normalisation filter through the social world is by determining what thoughts and practices are within the political context of PHAC's public health apparatus, with many exclusions being strategic and often subtle. While the disciplinary technique of exclusion may take many forms including discrimination, punishment, prohibition, segregation, elimination and omission (Jones 2000: 16), exclusion is not taken to such extremes on the PHAC website. Rather, the site incorporates the central characteristic shared by all forms of exclusion: not noticing that anything has actually been excluded.

On the WNV website specific forms of knowledge are the entities most often excluded. PHAC does not actively exclude ideas by discussing the concepts that are being rebuffed or by offering a rationalisation for the rejections: the existence of alternatives is just not mentioned. Therefore, although competing scientific and popular perspectives exist as to the threats related to the WNV, only one perspective – that of PHAC – is promoted. In order to accomplish such a task, PHAC has historically excluded information produced by organisations that reflect PHAC's basic conception of the virus yet oppose aspects of PHAC's control strategies, such as the use of specific chemicals in WNV treatment programmes. The possibility for debate is summarily dismissed through the centrality of texts on the website that describe the use of chemicals as an effective preventative strategy:

Insecticides, including larvicides and adulticides, are used to reduce the population of mosquitoes that could be capable of transmitting West Nile virus to humans. Larvicides may be used in First Nations communities where there is a medium or high risk of humans contracting West Nile virus. Adulticides are considered only as a last resort to prevent human infections in instances where there is significant risk to human health from West Nile virus and where prevention or mosquito control measures have failed or would clearly be inadequate to stop the spread of the virus. (First Nations and Inuit Health Branch 2005)

Although the sample text above points toward the possibility of problems with adulticides, notice how identification of a specific problem about adulticides is excluded. One effect of excluding other perspectives on the use of insecticides is that a dialogue between a range of experts in the fields of health, the environment, medicine and the Canadian public has been slow to develop and the knowledge accrued has been slow to be applied within the PHAC response. Practically, this also excludes the ways in which chemicals render outdoor spaces uninhabitable, whether the place is a neighbourhood that is toxic for a few hours after a fogging campaign or natural mosquito breeding habitats deemed to be high WNV infection zones summer after summer, which are, as a result, heavily sprayed with organophosphates. One of the cumulative effects of PHAC's exclusions is the production of a more profound philosophical extinguishment: the erosion of states of mind in which humans feel safe to move through the natural world without protective technologies (for example, insect repellents and specific kinds of clothing) and the banishment of an acceptance of vulnerability that can come from moving through natural environments (Gaard 1993, Merchant 1980, Sturgeon 1997) in which some entities, such as insects, cannot always be seen or controlled (Sandilands 1999).

Regulation
One way that PHAC proposes to diminish feelings of lack of safety and reduce the element of risk posed by the WNV is through the formal regulation of activities related to public health, many of which are legally binding and socially sanctioned, although they can be informally imposed as well as followed voluntarily. Discursive and non-discursive apparatuses such as social institutions, the architecture of buildings and social spaces, regulatory decisions, laws, administrative measures, scientific statements and technical processes all play a role in the enactment of regulation as a technique of power. Regulations are also generative in that they can be used to make particular substantive points or to cause specific material, political and social effects.

Importantly, the role of regulation in the production of the WNV is directly linked to the regulation of Canada's public healthcare delivery systems and is not explicitly related to the regulation of the general public. In other words, regulatory practices produce knowledge about the WNV by controlling the activities of knowledge producers in the context of PHAC. In the public health infrastructure, specific forms of regulation are an intrinsic part of the operations of PHAC. However, PHAC also uses the WNV pandemic to imbue these 'business as usual' regulatory practices with a renewed sense of urgency. Therefore, whether regulating insecticide use or the blood supply, it is the presence (or potential presence) of the WNV that PHAC uses to justify the development and exercise of many regulations and the attraction of additional resources pertaining to the efficacy of the agency's response to the WNV. To this end, PHAC not only generates the idea that the safety of Canadians necessitates the regulation of specific substances and institutional activities but also presents itself as the appropriate organisation to oversee these regulatory practices. On the page,

'What the Public Health Agency of Canada is doing', PHAC suggests that it is taking responsibility for the health and wellbeing of Canadians by performing a variety of supervisory and regulatory functions, including the following activities:

- Canada-wide surveillance for West Nile virus
- keeping Canada's blood system safe from West Nile virus
- testing for West Nile virus
- safe and effective pesticides and insect repellents
- keeping Canadians informed about new findings on West Nile virus
- working in collaboration with First Nations communities on reserves the Public Health Agency of Canada is coordinating a national approach to West Nile virus. (PHAC 2004c)

As this text implies, formal regulation is embedded within the structures, policies, mandates, and jurisdictions of the agencies involved in PHAC's WNV response. In this sense, PHAC's regulatory practices shape the possibilities of how the WNV can be understood and responded to in Canada. The Canadian public, however, is not formally regulated by the PHAC website nor are examples given of any formal punishment of Canadians engaged in 'risky' behaviour vis-à-vis the WNV: rather, people are encouraged voluntarily to take up the practices suggested by PHAC on the basis that the knowledge provided will be reason enough to participate in WNV prevention practices. PHAC's linking of regulatory activities with specific forms of knowledge, which it uses to justify the regulatory practices, fits with Foucault's (1980a) argument that, in power relations, power/knowledge plays an important role in the production of meaning and the organisation of the social world.

Conclusion

In June 2006 PHAC reframed its presentation of the WNV on its website. The WNV was demoted from a key epidemic concern, highlighted on the homepage, to one of a long list of infectious diseases under the PHAC remit. Substantively, however, the texts have remained largely the same, although in some cases new scientific information is presented and more speculative and sensationalised statements about the WNV risk have been removed. Shifts in the presentation of the WNV website over time embody the phenomenon of emergence and illustrate the ever-changing terrain of governmental constructions of EIDS, the kinds of governmental regulation and control regimes produced and the justifications given for their development.

Foucault observed that governmental activities often rationalise disciplinary practices by invoking the notion of the welfare of the population (1991: 100). A social constructionist analysis of the PHAC website has shown that PHAC's responses, produced through relations of power, are also the products of these same power/knowledge relations. This study has also contemplated issues of governmentality – not to reinscribe the view that disciplinary apparatuses are necessary because society is infused with risk (Beck 1992, 1995) or panic (Thompson 1998) but rather to show how specific configurations of relations of power produce notions like threat, risk and panic.

Emerging infectious diseases 'provide a valuable perspective for evaluating current trends' (Satcher 1995: 1). This chapter has questioned the normalisation of practices of regulation and administration as key features of contemporary public health approaches to infectious disease pandemics. In the nexus where the structures and institutions of (post) modern society develop 'risk cultures, political contingencies' and apparatuses of discipline (Turner 1997: xix), this study suggests that the fire-fighting orientation of public health responses should be complemented by prevention-based interventions that look upstream to the sources of emergences and the conditions that pre-exist emergence events. Epidemiological innovations and integrated public health responses to novel infectious diseases emergences based on a dynamic understanding of disease as produced in the nexus between human, microbial and ecological health may not claim to be able to completely regulate or eradicate EIDs but can and do produce knowledge around EID emergence processes that draw attention to the interplay between social, biological and ecological conditions which produce the conditions for a pandemic emergence.

Acknowledgements

I would like to thank Professors Pamela Moss, Martha McMahon and Bill Carroll of the University of Victoria for their counsel on the larger study I conducted and upon which this chapter is based.

References

Armstrong, D. (1997) Foucault and the sociology of health and illness: a prismatic reading. In Petersen, A. and Bunton, R. (eds) *Foucault, Health and Medicine*. London: Routledge.

Beck, U. (1992) *Risk Society: Towards a New Modernity*. London: Sage.

Beck, U. (1995) *Ecological Politics in an Age of Risk*. Cambridge: Polity Press.

Bendelow, G., Carpenter, M., Vautier, C. and Williams, S. (2002) Introduction: overcoming divisions: reflections on tradition, change, and critical continuity. In Carpenter, M., Vautier, C. and Williams, S. (eds) *Gender, Health and Healing: the Public/Private Divide*. London: Routledge.

Birke, L. (2002) Anchoring the head: the disappearing (biological) body. In Carpenter, M., Vautier, C. and Williams, S. (eds) *Gender, Health and Healing: the Public/Private Divide*. London: Routledge.

Busfield, J. (2002) The archaeology of psychiatric disorder: gender and disorders of thought, emotion and behaviour. In Carpenter, M., Vautier, C. and Williams, S. (eds) *Gender, Health and Healing: the Public/Private Divide*. London: Routledge.

Conrad, P. (1992) Medicalization and social control, *Annual Review of Sociology*, 18, 209–32.

Conrad, P. (ed.) (1995) *The Sociology of Health and Illness: Critical Perspectives* (7th edn). New York: Worth.

Ewald, F. (1991) *Insurance and risk*. In Burchell, G., Gordon, C. and Miller, P. (eds) *The Foucault Effect: Studies in Governmentality*. Chicago: University of Chicago Press.

First Nations and Inuit Health Branch (2005) First Nations and Innuit Health: West Nile virus. Available at http://www.hc-sc.gc.ca/fniah-spnia/diseases-maladies/wnv-vno/index-eng.php (accessed 11 September 2012).

Foucault, M. (1973) *The Order of Things: an Archaeology of the Human Sciences* (trans. A. Sheridan). New York: Vintage.

Foucault, M. (1980a) *The History of Sexuality, Volume 1: An Introduction*. New York: Vintage.

Foucault, M. (1980b) *Power and Knowledge: Selected Interviews and Other Writings, 1972–1977* (trans. C. Gordon, L. Marshall, J. Mephar and K. Sopher). New York: Pantheon.

Foucault, M. (1991) Governmentality. In Burchell, G., Gordon, C. and Miller, P (eds) *The Foucault Effect: Studies in Governmentality*. Chicago: University of Chicago Press.

Foucault, M. (1995) *Discipline and Punish: the Birth of the Prison* (2nd edn, trans. A. Sheridan). New York: Vintage.

Foucault, M. (2003) *The Birth of the Clinic* (1st edn). London: Routledge.

Gaard, G. (ed.) (1993) *Ecofeminism: Women, Animals, Nature*. Philadelphia: Temple University.

Gislason, M.K. (2010) Sounding a public health alarm: producing West Nile virus as a newly emerging infectious disease epidemic. In Mukherjea, A. (ed.) *Understanding Emerging Epidemics: Social and Political Approaches, Advances in Medical Sociology*. Bingley: Emerald.

Gonzales, J-P., Guiserix, M., Sauvage, F, Guitton, J-S., *et al.* (2010) Pathocenosis: a holistic approach to disease ecology, *EcoHealth*, 7, 2, 237–41.

Gore, J. (1995) On the continuity of power relations in pedagogy, *International Studies in Sociology of Education*, 5, 2, 165–88.

Gore, J. (1997) Who has the authority to speak about practice and how does it influence educational inquiry? Paper presented at the Australian Association for Research in Education Conference, Brisbane, 30 November to 4 December.

Gore, J. (2002) Micro-level techniques of power in the pedagogical production of class, race, gender and other relations. In Shapiro, H. and Shapiro, S. (eds) *Body Movements: Pedagogy, Politics and Social Change*. Cresskill: Hampton Press.

Health Canada (2006) West Nile virus – it's your health. Available at http://www.hc-sc.gc.ca/hl-vs/iyh-vsv/diseases-maladies/wnv-vno-eng.php (accessed 11 September 2012).

Jones, R. (2000) Digital rule punishment, control and technology, *Punishment and Society*, 2, 1, 5–22.

Laing, R. (1964) *Sanity, Madness and the Family, Volume 1: Families of Schizophrenics*. London: Tavistock.

McMichael, A. and Butler, C. (2007) Emerging health issues: the widening challenge for population health promotion, *Health Promotion International*, 21 (Supplement 1), 15–24.

Martin, E. (1994) *Flexible Bodies: the Role of Immunity in American Culture: from the Days of Polio to the Age of AIDS*. Boston: Beacon Press.

Merchant, C. (1980) *Death of Nature: Women, Ecology and the Scientific Revolution*. San Francisco: Harper and Row.

Moss, P. and Dyck, I. (2002) *Women, Body, Illness: Space and Identity in the Everyday Lives of Women with Chronic Illness*. Lanham: Rowman and Littlefield.

Mukherjea, A. (ed.) (2010) *Understanding Emerging Epidemics: Social and Political Approaches, Advances in Medical Sociology*. Bingley: Emerald.

Petersen, A. (1997) Risk, governance and the new public health. In Petersen, A. and Bunton, R. (eds), *Foucault, Health and Medicine*. London: Rutledge.

Petersen, A. and Bunton, R. (eds) (1997) *Foucault, Health and Medicine*. London: Routledge.

Petersen, A. and Lupton, D. (1997) *The New Public Health: Health and Self in the Age of Risk*. London: Sage.

Price-Smith, A. (2001) *Plagues and Politics: Infectious Disease and International Policy*. Basingstoke: Palgrave.

Public Health Agency of Canada (PHAC) (2004a) Surveillance, education, prevention and response. Available at http://www.phac-aspc.gc.ca/wn-no/surveillance-eng.php#5 (accessed 11 September 2012).

PHAC (2004a) General overview. Available at: http://www.phac-aspc.gc.ca/wn-no/gen-eng.php (accessed 11 September 2012).

PHAC (2004b) What the government of Canada is doing. Available at: http://www.phac-aspc.gc.ca/wn-no/role_e.html (accessed 11 September 2012).

PHAC (2009) West Nile virus – protect yourself! Available at http://www.phac-aspc.gc.ca/wn-no/index-eng.php (accessed 11 September 2012).

PHAC (2012) Protect yourself and your family. Available at http://www.phac-aspc.gc.ca/wn-no/protect-proteger-eng.php (accessed 11 September 2012).

Rouse, J. (1994) Power/Knowledge. In Gutting. G. (ed.) *The Cambridge Companion to Foucault*. Cambridge: Cambridge University Press.

Sandilands, C. (1999) *The Good Natured Feminist: Ecofeminism and the Quest for Democracy*. Minneapolis: University of Minnesota Press.

Satcher, D. (1995) Emerging infections: getting ahead of the curve, *Emerging Infectious Diseases*, 1, 1, 1–6.

Senellart, M. (ed) (2007) *Michel Foucault: Security, Territory, Population.* Basingstoke: Palgrave Macmillan.

Shilling, C. (2005) *The Body in Culture, Technology and Society.* London: Sage.

Stephenson, N. and Jamieson, M. (2009) Securitising health: Australian newspaper coverage of pandemic influenza, *Sociology of Health & Illness*, 31, 4, 525–39.

Sturgeon, N. (1997) *Ecofeminist Natures: Race, Gender, Feminist Theory and Political Action.* New York: Routledge.

Tausig, M., Selgelid, M., Subedi, S. and Subedi, J. (2006) Taking sociology seriously: a new approach to the bioethical problems of infectious disease, *Sociology of Health & Illness*, 28, 6, 838–49.

Thompson, K. (1998) *Moral Panics.* London: Routledge.

Timmermans, S and Haas, S. (2008) Towards a sociology of disease, *Sociology of Health & Illness*, 30, 5, 659–76.

Turner, B. (1997) Forward: From governmentality to risk: some reflections on Foucault's contribution to medical sociology. In Petersen, A. and Bunton, R. (eds) *Foucault, Health and Medicine.* London: Routledge.

Waltner-Toews, D. (2007) *The Chickens Fight Back: Pandemic Panics and Deadly Diseases That Jump from Animals to Humans.* Vancouver: Greystone.

Washer, P. (2010) *Emerging Infectious Diseases and Society.* Basingstoke: Palgrave Macmillan.

World Health Organization (2005) WHO global influenza preparedness plan: The role of the WHO and recommendations for national measures before and during pandemics http://www.who.int/csr/resources/publications/influenza/en/WHO_CDS_CSR_GIP_2005_5.pdf (accessed 3 September 2012).

4

Who's worried about turkeys? How 'organisational silos' impede zoonotic disease surveillance

Colin Jerolmack

Introduction

In 2009, the 'swine flu' (H1N1) reached pandemic proportions, killing hundreds, hospitalising thousands, and frightening millions. Like the 'avian flu' (H5N1), H1N1 originated in animals. Though H1N1 remains far less lethal to humans than H5N1, H1N1 reached a milestone by mutating to the point where it can pass between humans without an animal host. The mutation and re-assortment of flu strains as they jump across species raises the spectre of a 'super virus' with H1N1's transmissibility and H5N1's virulence.

Several months after H1N1 became a pandemic, it was discovered for the first time in birds. This raised the possibility of the virus recombining with flu genes from its new hosts – turkeys – to produce a more lethal strain. Yet the *New York Times* reported that 'health officials were not particularly alarmed' about the spread of H1N1 to birds. Dr. Anthony Fauci, who oversaw the US government's clinical trials of the H1N1 vaccine, declared 'it's widespread in humans, so who cares if it's in turkeys?' Although 'you could dream up a variety of scenarios' in which the spread of H1N1 to birds could produce a deadlier flu strain, Fauci said, 'we have enough H1N1 to worry about without worrying about turkeys'. He concluded that turkey infection is 'a Department of Agriculture issue' (McNeil 2009: A10).

Because 'human and animal diseases [are] treated as separate entities' (Kahn *et al.* 2007: 11), human health organisations seldom monitor animal health or consider it relevant to their institutional prerogatives – a truth Dr. Fauci plainly revealed. Just as troubling, I find a similar organisational 'silo effect' among the various animal health agencies. While diseases disregard boundaries between species and socially constructed categories of animals (e.g. pets, wildlife), organisations do not. To explain this phenomenon, this chapter examines how agents that monitor human and animal health – for example, employees of the Department of Health (DOH), the United States Department of Agriculture (USDA), the Department of Wildlife, and the Centers for Disease Control (CDC) – each operate within a distinct organisational culture. I show how the mission, jurisdiction, and institutionalised practices of each bureaucracy can constrain members' ability to successfully respond to emerging infectious diseases (EIDs) that flout organisational borders. My attribution of agency to diseases is literal (Latour 1988) – it is the proliferation of 'hybrid' (species-jumping) EIDs that creates the relational problem I call organisational silos (Figure 1).

Pandemics and Emerging Infectious Diseases: The Sociological Agenda, First Edition. Edited by Robert Dingwall, Lily M. Hoffman and Karen Staniland. Chapters © 2013 The Authors. Book Compilation © 2013 Foundation for the Sociology of Health & Illness / John Wiley & Sons Ltd.

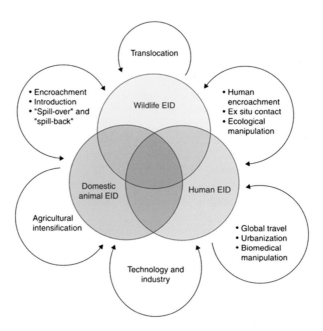

Figure 1 *The host–pathogen 'ecological continuum' for zoonotic EIDs. Arrows denote some of the key drivers of EIDs. From Daszak et al. 2000. Reprinted with permission from AAAS*

EIDs are defined by the US Institute of Medicine as 'infectious diseases that have recently increased in incidence or geographical range, recently been discovered, or are caused by newly evolved pathogens' (Cunningham 2005: 1214). Over 60 per cent of EIDs are zoonotic, meaning that they can be transmitted from animals to humans (Jones *et al.* 2008). The contemporary prevalence of zoonoses is related to changes in human ecology (Jones *et al.* 2008): ecosystem disruption and urbanisation (which can cause animal viruses to spill into human settlements and produce unsanitary 'mega slums'), intensive livestock production (which concentrates disease vectors), and global travel and trade (which quickly spreads pathogens around the world).

Human health agencies should care about turkeys because the surveillance of animal diseases can prevent the emergence of human diseases. The bureaucratic and cultural divide between veterinary and human medicine is one of the principal problems hampering efforts to contain zoonoses (Gibbs and Anderson 2009). While the emergent 'One Health' movement and the recent reorganisation of the CDC reflect an awareness that human and animal health are interdependent, fewer people seem aware of the analogous divides that exist among animal health practitioners. Socially constructed categories such as 'livestock' and 'wildlife' have been encoded into mutually exclusive agencies (e.g. the USDA, Wildlife Services) whose responses to zoonoses are shaped by inter-organisational struggles over jurisdictions, resources and reputations. While controlling 'hybrid' diseases requires hybrid knowledge and interagency cooperation, the typical division of labour in epidemiology propagates a silo effect rather than systems thinking. Interagency collaboration is often *ad hoc* or overly reliant on charismatic leaders and interpersonal relations (Leslie and McQuiston 2007).

Sociologists of health should also care about turkeys, lest they reify the dualism between human and animal health that has hampered efforts to contain zoonoses. The concept of organisational silos provides us with a useful way to think about the relational difficulties that arise when disparate disciplines and organisations converge on 'hybrid' problems like zoonoses.

Methods

Most of this chapter's data derive from semi-structured interviews (1–2 hours long) and follow-up emails with state and federal epidemiologists, veterinarians, and physicians carried out in 2008–2009 (N = 15). Except for two phone interviews, all interviews were face-to-face; ten were audio-recorded. Rather than snowball sampling, I selected experienced 'key informants' who occupied similar structural positions in animal and human health agencies and who seemed positioned to 'think in terms of the organisation' and report upon its day-to-day operations (Seidler 1974: 817). Because concerns over 'biosecurity' made direct observation unviable, I asked informants to describe their routines, disease events they responded to, and their relations to other agencies. Eleven of my informants worked in human and animal health agencies or divisions located in a mid-sized Northeastern US city.[1] These include: the state Department of Health; the city Public Health Commission; the state Department of Agriculture; the regional division of the US Department of Agriculture; and the local Animal Rescue League. While no singleton perfectly embodies an organisation, interviewing key decision-makers in one city allowed me to see how they interpreted their organisation's prerogatives and worked together on local disease events.

One of the remaining four informants was the director of the CDC's Geographic Medicine and Health Promotion Branch. Of the last three, one worked in another state's livestock health agency and two worked in that state's human health agency. I also spoke with more than a dozen doctors and veterinarians, and attended sessions, at an all-day professional conference on zoonoses; and I attended a panel discussion hosted by Dr. Michael Greger, the Humane Society's director of Public Health and Animal Agriculture and the author of a book about the bird flu (2006). My conclusions are also informed by epidemiological reports issued by the organisations in question, and by case studies of disease events.

Institutional interaction and organisational culture

All formal organisations contain 'enduring elements of social life – institutions – that have a profound effect on the thoughts, feelings, and behaviour of individual and collective actors' (Lawrence and Suddaby 2006: 216). Institutions are 'rules and shared meanings . . . that define social relationships . . . and guide interaction by giving actors *cognitive frames* to interpret the behavior of others' (Fligstein 2001: 108). Organisations define the goals, the forms of valued competence and knowledge, and the avenues by which their members can achieve desired goals. Over time these supra-individual understandings become encoded in 'standardized interaction sequences' (Lawrence and Suddaby 2006: 216). This is how institutions emerge. The constellation of institutions that hang together in an organisation, the 'beliefs, behaviors, and customs shared by all members', can be conceptualised as an organisational culture (Fine 1979: 734). As members strategically respond to the exigencies of their

social role, they routinely rely on organisational culture to orient their behaviour and interpret others' behaviour (Vaughan 1996). In turn, their situated practices and sense-making
also contribute to the maintenance – and sometimes transformation – of the very culture
they draw upon to act.

'Institutional thinking' can 'reproduce characteristic definitions of and solutions to social
problems' (Irvine 2003: 550) because organisational members may only consider a solution
'right' 'if it sustains the institutional thinking' that is already in their minds (Douglas 1986:
4). Although actors can creatively navigate within their organisational field (DiMaggio
1988), institutional categories of thought may be so taken-for-granted or 'naturalised' that
they escape members' awareness.

If the realm of infectious diseases is a map, then agencies like the USDA or a state DOH
each patrol a specific territory whose borders are both geographic (e.g. state or federal) and
substantive (e.g. animal or human health). Each territorial unit has its own bureaucracy
and mission (e.g. protecting livestock or wildlife); and each cultivates unique habits of
thought and action – an 'institutional fingerprint' (Drew and Heritage 1992) – that codify
the organisation. These agencies, then, 'concern themselves with specific aspects of nature'
while excluding 'other aspects of nature which may be judged to be peripheral or only
loosely connected to the concerns of [the] regulatory institution' (Brown and Michael 2004:
208–9). So how do these agencies respond to 'hybrid' natural phenomena (i.e., zoonotic
EIDs) that ignore borders?

I argue that organisational cultures become silos when the factors that make agencies so
well adapted to their particular set of problems breed an inflexibility that hinders tackling
inter-jurisdictional or 'hybrid' problems. The cultures of two institutions may even clash;
detailed below, the Department of Wildlife may stand in direct opposition to the Department
of Agriculture when an EID circulates between livestock and wildlife. Rather than cooperat-
ing, each side may rush to blame the other for a disease outbreak as it seeks to protect
animals in its jurisdiction. Conceiving of animal and human health agencies as organisations
with distinct cultures helps clarify why they so often lack the flexibility needed to success-
fully respond to species-jumping EIDs. These 'hybrid' diseases transgress and blur categories that organisations have worked to segregate and naturalise (e.g. 'wildlife', 'livestock').
Addressing the systemic character of zoonoses may challenge the *raison d'être* of traditional
animal and human health organisations.

While many sociologists study within an organisation, the silo effect metaphor draws
attention to the relational problem of institutional thinking across organisations. It is the
emergence of new 'hybrid' problems (e.g. zoonotic EIDs) that makes organisational cultures
function as silos – the notion of organisational silos denotes a lack of mutual understanding,
common goals, and communication between agencies whose concerns are systemically
linked.

Priorities, jurisdictions and silos

Dave Spencer, the director of the Animal Health Division at the state's Department of
Agriculture, is intent on protecting agriculture. 'We're here to support anyone doing farming
[and] keeping animals', he told me. 'We consider even somebody with a horse in their
backyard as agriculture, and we want people to continue keeping animals on their property'.
This means that Spencer defended animal caretakers facing 'not in my backyard' complaints
from neighbours and the DOH. 'If it's done right', he believed, 'it should be OK if it's in
everyone's backyard'.

Spencer's attitude is not surprising given that he works for the Department of Agriculture. But what matters is how his position shapes his response to diseases and other organisations. He mentioned the case of a swine farm near a residential area in which credible complaints about the improper disposal of faeces led local legislators to consider passing a new law that would force the farmer to move. The situation, Spencer recalled, pitted the Department of Agriculture against 'the DOH, the Environmental Protection Agency, and a whole bunch of other federal and state agencies'. The case remained unresolved, but Spencer made a veiled threat: 'I don't know who's going to remove his animals. It's certainly not something we're going to do'.

Spencer saw shutting down the farm as antithetical to his agency's mission, even if the state told him to. He framed the affair as typical of the hostility between local health boards and animal caretakers. Because of the state's 'home rule', each town can create distinct laws regarding livestock. Spencer felt that these boards do not value the role of agriculture in a community and overestimate the disease risk. In response, his agency musters resources to back farmers when they come into conflict with agencies and neighbours, and to preserve farms by subsidising land easements. He calls many neighbour complaints 'overblown', claiming they 'always go for the jugular' by whipping up fears of viruses like H5N1.

Spencer sometimes chafed at disease response guidelines handed down to him from state and federal governments. 'We got a positive [flu result] on one of our routine surveillance tests' of a poultry farm, Spencer complained, and 'we were required to contact the USDA right away because of the pandemic Asian strain'. Spencer added, 'It seems a little silly because there was no clinical illness on the property, and the strain came back something pretty common'. Though the strain was non-zoonotic, he said that the requirement to notify 'the feds' prompted Japan to ban imports from the state. He was annoyed that an 'automatic rule', which to him was an 'overreaction' that should not apply to this case, had cost state poultry farmers so dearly.

In Spencer's eyes, it was 'hard to justify' reporting the flu strain to the USDA. He shared a similar story about how a mundane flu strain that appeared in some poultry led him to inform the town's board of health. 'Before we knew it, they were putting out a press release and scaring the crap out of everyone'. He said this result made him hesitant to contact local health boards in future cases of non-zoonotic bird flu outbreaks: 'That's not necessarily a good thing, but it's an unfortunate side effect of something that went wrong last time'. These days, Spencer said he passes on information about disease events to the state DOH and leaves it to them to tell local health boards. 'If somebody screws up', he shrugged, 'at least we can blame the [DOH]'.

Though Spencer mentioned a few times that he cooperated with other agencies, on the whole he seemed distrustful – particularly of human health agencies. In the end, he told me, 'We work a lot more with animal control programs than with boards of health. The town boards of health are the ones we have the least communication with'. While the USDA was his closest ally, Spencer still accused this federal agency of occasionally meddling in the state's affairs.

Spencer was looking out for his agency's reputation, not just farmers. This is strikingly revealed in his confession of using the state DOH as a buffer and occasional scapegoat. He viewed this as an adaptive response to prior situations in which other agencies, advancing their agendas, left him 'high and dry'. Spencer refused to blame any consequential disease outbreaks on livestock, noting only the existence of flu strains that posed no risk to people. He always came back to wildlife when I asked him about the main sources or vectors for zoonoses.

Spencer's counterpart in the Northeast division of the USDA's Animal and Plant Health Inspection Service (APHIS), Steven Clinton, had a similar outlook. APHIS is charged with 'protecting American agriculture . . . [and] improving agricultural productivity and competitiveness'.[2] Clinton said that his primary responsibilities included monitoring imports and exports of live animals and 'biomedical products' – particularly at ports of entry to the US – that could introduce new zoonoses. He lamented that, because 'the agricultural footprint in [the Northeast] is smaller than elsewhere, we tend not to see it as critical to the economy or food needs'. He added that there were also a lot of rumours and 'unreasonable amplifications of risk' surrounding livestock diseases. Clinton saw regional farmers as an embattled class of people needing muscular protection.

Clinton argued that the 'single biggest threat for disease' comes from 'wildlife intermingling with domestic livestock'. He told me, 'You can't control the birds' and he rightly pointed out that ducks are flu incubators. If the bird flu – which Clinton called the top priority of his agency – becomes pandemic in humans, he told me, it will come from waterfowl. Given these realities, he was frustrated at how little money is allotted to his agency and others that monitor animals: 'The CDC's strategic national stockpile for the flu is a half billion dollars, but the veterinary stockpile for animal disease is about three million'.

Clinton and Spencer both placed the blame for most zoonoses on wildlife; and neither of them spoke about partnerships with state or federal wildlife agencies. The gap between these two worlds seemed even wider than the gap between agriculture and public health. Whether or not a disease originated in wildlife, zoonoses routinely circulate between livestock and wildlife before they jump to humans (Davis 2005). Thus, it seems troubling that communication between these wildlife and livestock agencies seemed to be lacking. Regardless of where a disease came from, both sides should be interested in gleaning as much information as possible and enacting surveillance systems to track its circulation. Because of the rapid mutation that can occur as flu strains undergo genetic re-assortment in animal hosts, both sides need to be aware of what the virus is doing inside animal bodies that are outside their agency's jurisdiction.

Even though veterinarian Rebecca Black from the state DOH had a working relationship with Dave Spencer in the Department of Agriculture, she did not share his perspective on zoonoses. Although Dr. Black emphasised that this was 'just my opinion', she said on more than one occasion that 'most wildlife do not pose a disease risk to us'. She insinuated that economic interests sometimes made agricultural agencies allergic to acknowledging disease outbreaks among livestock (see Davis 2005). Black admitted that the relationship between the DOH and the Department of Agriculture was strained because of this clash of interests and perspectives, and that this sometimes meant that the DOH did not receive information on circulating diseases in animals that may become a problem for humans later on. Because flu strains can mutate quickly, Black considered even non-zoonotic bird flu outbreaks among poultry to be significant and relevant public health information – the Department of Agriculture did not.

Dr. Michael Greger,[3] the director of Public Health and Animal Agriculture at the Humane Society, was cynical about why agricultural agencies often eschew cooperation with outside agencies: livestock, he said, cause most EIDs. The author of a book that blames concentrated animal feeding operations (CAFOs) for the looming H5N1 pandemic, during a panel discussion on the bird flu Greger described the dangers of 'warehousing' animals: having so many 'nose to nose' allows viruses and bacteria to develop and mutate quickly as they pass between hosts; and, as farmers rush to prevent diseases with antimicrobials, mutating diseases select for virulence as they adapt to antimicrobial regimes. While some of the diseases incubating in livestock may have originated in wildlife, they typically remain chronic but not particularly virulent in the wild. Crowding is the key to becoming zoonotic – and deadly (see also Davis 2005).

Dr. Greger's hard line on agriculture fits squarely within the Humane Society's mission. By spotlighting the crowded conditions of CAFOs, Greger used concerns over avian flu to bring attention to inhumane animal treatment. Yet Greger's claims echo the CDC and the World Health Organization, which both said that the killing of wildlife across Asia in response to H5N1 was 'counterproductive' and argued instead for regulating CAFOs (Waltner-Toews 2007). Nina Marano,[4] a zoonotic disease expert at the CDC, told me that 'most of the outbreaks have occurred through interaction with domestic poultry'. Another example: though poultry farmers singled out wild birds called cattle egrets as the source of a 2004 flu outbreak in California, the egrets tested negative – it turned out that contaminated egg containers circulating between farms were the culprit (McNeil 2004). Such cases pit wildlife proponents against livestock proponents, as their interests and reputational integrity depend on evading culpability.

Though Rebecca Black felt that wildlife posed less of a zoonotic threat than livestock, as an agent of the DOH – which prioritises human health – she also clashed with the Department of Wildlife: 'Often, our interests bring us into conflict. For example, a few cases of a disease being transmitted from animals to humans – say, Lyme disease – may be considered a big problem by the DOH and a reason for action' [such as culling wildlife]. 'However, [the Department of Wildlife] may say that there's not much of a threat or need for action because there are so many interactions of humans and these animals and so few of them have resulted in transmission'. As a veterinarian, Black said she is more sensitive to balancing these concerns than her colleagues; but, as a DOH employee, she sometimes felt beholden to institutional mandates to exterminate populations of wild animals that she may not personally think are necessary.

Rebecca Black spoke more about relationships with the Department of Wildlife and other groups engaged in feral / wild animal control than about the Department of Agriculture. This is likely because rabies is the zoonose that the DOH pays most attention to; this lethal virus routinely relies on wild animals as a reservoir and can find its way to humans through bites from stray and feral cats and dogs. But the fact that the only zoonose Black mentioned without my prodding was rabies reflected the reality that the DOH did little regular surveillance of other zoonoses.

The importance of the things left unsaid was even more apparent when I spoke to Dr. Vanessa Sanders, the director of the Infectious Disease Bureau of the city Public Health Commission. Sanders made clear to me that, while her 'home rule' city board communicates with state agencies and must abide by certain state and federal regulations, 'we are not beholden to them'. When I asked Sanders to describe a zoonose that she responded to, she mentioned a recent outbreak of salmonella. She noticed that many of the infected people had Asian surnames, and she believed that the pathogen came from two live poultry markets in Chinatown. What I found telling was that, in Sanders' lengthy discussion of this outbreak, she did not mention any communication with veterinary medicine agencies. While the Disease Bureau's response to salmonella followed protocol, it did not turn to the Department of Agriculture, the USDA, or any other agencies involved in animal health for help or information. Nor did it share information with them. When I asked how to address the problem of salmonella and other germs from animals in Chinatown, Sanders mentioned the need to change residents' cultural practices but neglected veterinary medicine solutions.

When I turned to the topic of other zoonoses such as Lyme disease and West Nile virus,[5] again Sanders only spoke about the human dimension. It became clear that the Disease

Bureau remained in a reactive position regarding zoonoses: it did not regularly communicate with animal agencies or analyse surveillance data on disease outbreaks in animals, but instead responded with medical and educational campaigns once one or more people became infected. The city's Disease Bureau seemed even more insulated from the world of veterinary medicine than the state DOH, perhaps because the DOH employed a veterinarian.

The US response to West Nile virus is instructive of how human and animal health agencies can exist in organisational silos. Crows started dying in New York in May of 1999, and a veterinary clinic that analysed the carcasses noted neurological symptoms. By August, a Queens hospital had admitted eight people displaying similar neurological symptoms. After the hospital contacted the DOH, the patients were wrongly diagnosed with St. Louis encephalitis; three later died. Meanwhile, the chief of the Bronx Zoo's pathology department, Tracy McNamara, found the same symptoms in some zoo birds. She immediately suspected a link between the human and animal sicknesses, yet if the disease was encephalitis it should not have killed the birds. The CDC and the local DOH, feeling secure with their diagnoses, ignored McNamara's offer to share her findings and her requests to obtain information on the human cases (Kahn 2007). Indeed, Clinton (USDA) and Black (DOH) both told me that agencies 'always respond to the last crisis', which can blind them to new information.

It was largely McNamara's tenacity that led to the discovery of West Nile. After the CDC and the New York DOH rebuffed her, she sent specimens to a friend at the US Army Medical Research Institute of Infectious Diseases – which overturned the encephalitis diagnosis. Henry Walasek, an epidemiologist who works for the city's Animal Rescue League, told me it was a 'wake up call'. He was disgusted at the 'dumb luck' that led to the diagnosis: 'They just found this virus by accident, because a zoo pathologist happened to notice something wasn't right with dead crows. And then, only because she pursued [it], lo and behold there was West Nile'. The fact that its discovery hinged on one dogged veterinarian did not bode well for zoonotic surveillance systems. By the time West Nile was found, it was endemic; and the trouble McNamara had in getting the CDC and the DOH to listen to her indicated the lack of cooperation and data sharing between human and animal medicine (see also Leslie and McQuiston 2007).

Though the discovery of West Nile was greeted with alarm and massive pesticide sprays, it did not usher in a sea change regarding zoonotic surveillance and communications across states and agencies. Clinton from the USDA complained to me that the West Nile fiasco 'faded away from public consciousness' without changing 'business as usual'. 'Most surveillance systems', a *Health Affairs* article states, are still inadequate, 'passive, and disease specific' (Morse 2007: 1070). 'While surveillance of humans helps identify infectious disease threats', opines a physician in an article reflecting on the legacy of West Nile, 'we should budget more money for wildlife surveillance, as it is from this reservoir that many novel – and potentially deadly – infectious agents will emerge' (Kahn 2007: 68).

Forging systemic connections

Lessons are being learned. Yet the fractured landscape of human and animal health agencies stifles efforts to implement them. When I asked Dave Spencer from the state Department of Agriculture what rules governed keeping livestock in suburban and urban areas, he smirked, 'There aren't any. Most of the rules, if a town decides to make them, are on a town-by-town basis'. This makes it nearly impossible for the state to implement standards for reporting and monitoring disease. As shown above, 'home rule' can create tension and distrust between local and state agencies – not a good basis for coordination. And it practically guarantees both gaps in surveillance and redundancy across locales.

Though home rule in the state I studied may be extreme, it highlights a problem that goes up to the federal level. As a professor of virology notes, 'There are 200 different government offices and programmes responding to five zoonotic diseases' (Gibbs 2005: 679). After remarking that various disease surveillance systems are not linked, he adds, 'There is no coordinated effort or single agency with 'command and control' responsibility' over 'animal and public health' (Gibbs 2005: 679). Akin to nation-states, the more semi-autonomous animal and human health agencies found on the public health map, the harder it is to foster cooperation. Also like nation-states, sharply defined borders enable the proliferation of unique cultures – organisational outlooks and customary practices.[6] These cultures can become silos that bind actors to internal organisational prerogatives and constrain creative responses to EIDs and cross-agency collaboration. The growing incidence of EIDs, and the few public health successes that resulted from experimentation, should embolden health practitioners to chart a new direction.

Recently, the CDC has made emerging zoonoses a priority. A person at the forefront of its efforts is Dr. Nina Marano. She became director of the Geographic Medicine and Health Promotion Branch when it was founded in 2006. 'It was created', she told me, 'in recognition of the fact that emerging diseases – particularly since 1999 – have been zoonotic in origin, starting with West Nile and going forward to SARS and influenza'. Marano said that the CDC recognised that its traditional division along 'specific disease lines' – for example, parasites – no longer made sense when, in fact, all of the diseases came from animals. The CDC also recognised the need to do 'a better job of building relationships with the veterinary world'.

Marano, as a veterinarian, was put in charge of a division that tracked the flows of both humans (as travellers) and animals (as they are imported or exported). The idea is that the likely pathway of a new EID to the US is on a plane. Whether it comes from an animal or human was not paramount to her – the result is the same. This approach allowed Marano to focus on following diseases as they cross borders and species. On a daily basis, she said she talked to and analysed data from US Customs, Fish and Wildlife, the USDA, local Departments of Health, and so on. Marano's job was not to specialise or carve out a jurisdiction – she aimed to be at the centre of a Venn diagram of human and animal health agencies.

The CDC is absorbing the lessons of prior EIDs and constructing far-reaching and flexible departments whose hybrid structures mirror the hybridity of the viruses they track (cf. Brown and Michael 2004). In 2007, it reorganised some of its oldest divisions under the newly created National Center for Zoonotic, Vector-Borne, and Enteric Diseases (ZVED), whose mission is to 'understand, prevent, control and – where possible – eliminate infectious diseases within a larger ecological context [that] includes humans, animals, and plants interacting in the complex, ever-changing natural environment'.[7] Rather than 'always responding to the last crisis', ZVED aims to forecast and head off the next one. This means being open to novel interpretations of data and not stopping at the most likely diagnosis – a lesson learned when health agencies mistook West Nile for encephalitis. It was only through dismantling traditional departments that the CDC could break up ossified organisational cultures and supplant the silo effect with systems thinking.

Though the CDC interfaces with state agencies, these organisations have a lot of autonomy in the US federalist system (Morse 2007). While scarce funding may be the culprit, states severely lag behind the CDC in reorganising agencies and blurring jurisdictions so that they can take an holistic approach to zoonoses. It is hard to imagine a ZVED-like structure arising out of the Balkanised bureaucratic map in states like the one I studied. In its absence, members often seem to hold strong allegiances to their particular organisation and its jurisdictional neck of the woods. Bureaucratic epidemiological divisions along socially constructed categories of animals, like livestock and wildlife, seem particularly obdurate and outmoded. While zoonoses pay no heed to whether their hosts are designated as 'wild' or 'domestic' animals, the existence of agencies solely dedicated to the health of animals that fall within one of these designations has the effect of naturalising such categorical distinctions and fostering a sense of apathy or even antagonism towards categories of animals that fall outside an agency's purview.

However, the reaction to rabies in the state I studied indicates that cooperation on the state level is possible. In response to a spike in reported rabies cases in the 1990s, the state Department of Agriculture worked closely with, and trained, livestock inspectors and veterinarians in hundreds of towns. Spencer said his office was talking with the state Department of Wildlife and the DOH 'at least five times a day' during the height of the scare. He was also regularly in touch with the CDC. The Department of Wildlife took the lead on trapping and testing wild animals and promptly shared all findings with the DOH. Rebecca Black, the veterinarian at the DOH, explained that the state committed a lot of money to rabies, which enabled the DOH to oversee the response to rabies across myriad agencies, stockpile costly post-exposure prophylaxes, and launch an extensive public education campaign. Because pets are usually the bridge between rabid wildlife and people, health agencies reached out to animal control officers. Henry Walasek (Animal Rescue League), who was often left out of the public health loop, said that his agency was central to the rabies response because it often rescued stray pets that could be rabid.

Rabies is a paradigmatic example of the successful alignment of priorities and action among the myriad agencies responsible for human and animal health – both in the state I studied and nationally (see Leslie and McQuiston 2007). Interagency advisory committees smoothed coordination. Vaccination rates of pets went up, and the number of wildlife-to-pet/human infections steadily declined after 1994. We can draw important lessons from the rabies response, but its success may not be easily replicable because of insufficient resources. Several of the epidemiologists I spoke with were actually frustrated with the time and energy the state devoted to rabies because they believed it was partly driven by a desire to allay what Walasek called the public's 'fear and hysteria'. Though the objective risk of contracting rabies was very low, they argued, the public's subjective risk assessment was off the charts (see Slovic 1987).

Is sustained inter-agency interaction only possible in the face of a panic-inducing disease? Agencies must find ways to keep lines of communication open in between frightful disease events, and human health agencies need to get interested in zoonoses other than rabies. Fittingly, a representative from the 'One Health Commission' recently attended the 'World Rabies Day' conference to highlight how rabies is simply one of many zoonoses that can only be controlled through the cooperation of veterinary and human medicine. The One Health Commission discourages over-specialisation among clinicians and agencies, reminding us, 'The convergence of people, animals, and our environment has created a new dynamic in which the health of each group is inextricably interconnected' (King 2008: 260).

On the ground level, there are some cases of systemic linkages. The American Veterinary Medical Association and the American Medical Association now organise 'One Health' forums that allow practising physicians and veterinarians – who are, in effect, at the forefront of disease surveillance and treatment efforts – to compare notes on disease events and trends. I went to one of these conferences in Rhode Island, entitled 'Pets, People, and

Pathogens: Emerging Diseases', which was well attended and featured a wide range of panels that stimulated questions and fruitful discussions between veterinarians and physicians. It was apparent that these two worlds are still learning how to interact, but there seemed to be genuine enthusiasm for the endeavour and – perhaps most importantly – the formation of personal ties that could develop into social networks for circulating information and tracking emerging trends.

The internet may be an invaluable tool of grassroots efforts, as clinicians take advantage of Listservs like ProMed to quickly disseminate reports about new infections – no matter where in the world they occur. Perhaps, with both clinicians and the CDC increasingly embracing 'One Health', they can pressure state agencies from both sides into adapting to the EID threats of the 21st century. Perhaps paradoxically, this study highlights that they may face more resistance within the realm of animal health than across the human-animal divide.

Conclusion

This chapter used insights from organisational sociology to understand why human and animal health agencies have had trouble changing their practices in response to species-jumping infectious diseases. Although each agency's institutionalised habits of thought and action may have been relatively well-adapted to addressing the diseases that traditionally concerned each organisation, they constrain members from building the inter-organisational and interdisciplinary bridges required to manage the latest 'hybrid' diseases. It is for this reason that zoonotic EIDs can be said to produce the silo effect – the standard epidemiological division of labour has become anachronistic as ecological disruptions and globalisation enable diseases to freely jump across species, borders, and categories of animals. The degree of institutional change necessary to address new zoonoses, I have implied, may be unthinkable to some animal and health agencies because the institutionalised frames that their members employ to interpret the problem are so taken-for-granted that they escape members' awareness. For instance, no species is inherently 'livestock' or 'wildlife'. But such categories have become naturalised and serve as the foundation for the division of labour in animal health. Agency members interpret certain diseases as 'livestock diseases' or 'wildlife diseases', and they view categories of animals outside their purview as irrelevant to their institutional prerogatives. Consequently, there is little sense of mutual understanding and common goals – and thus little coordination – across these various organisations. They may even see each other as adversaries as they struggle to protect their interests, jurisdictions, and reputations. While sociological studies typically focus within an organisation, I have introduced the concept of 'organisational silos' to capture the relational dilemmas that arise when a 'hybrid' problem systemically links together agencies with disparate organisational cultures.

While more and more health practitioners recognise the problematic divide between human and animal health, my exploratory findings indicate that there can be severe and antagonistic divisions within the realm of animal health. This seems to be an important but neglected problem of zoonotic disease surveillance and health policy. Finally, social scientists are also guilty of neglecting the connection between human and animal health (Rock et al. 2009). Zoonoses promise to dominate the domain of infectious diseases this century. If we seek to produce scholarship that medical practitioners can use to improve public health, we would do well to follow these diseases – and the agencies tracking them – into the non-human realm.

Acknowledgements

This research was made possible by a fellowship from the Robert Wood Johnson Scholars in Health Policy Research Program and was carried out while I was in residence at Harvard University.

Notes

1 Unless otherwise noted, names are pseudonyms (upon request). To ensure my informants' anonymity and respect their concerns about biosecurity, I also mask the city and state.
2 http://www.aphis.usda.gov/.
3 Not a pseudonym.
4 Not a pseudonym.
5 West Nile virus, a recent arrival to the US, is passed from birds to people via mosquito bites.
6 The nation-state comparison is more than an analogy – the intergovernmental World Organisation for Animal Health operates with the express goal of reducing the international silo effect by coordinating and standardizing zoonotic disease reporting across national borders.
7 http://www.cdc.gov/nczved/about.html.

References

Brown, N. and Michael, M. (2004) Risky creatures: Institutional species boundary change in biotechnology regulation, *Health, Risk and Society*, 6, 3, 207–22.
Cunningham, A.A. (2005) A walk on the wild side – emerging wildlife diseases, *British Medical Journal*, 331, 7527, 1214–5.
Daszak, P., Cunningham, A.A. and Hyatt, A.D. (2000) Emerging infectious diseases of wildlife: Threats to biodiversity and human health, *Science*, 287, 5452, 443–9.
Davis, M. (2005) *The Monster at Our Door: The Global Threat of Avian Flu*. New York: Owl Books.
DiMaggio, P.J. (1988) Interest and agency in institutional theory. In Zucker, L.G. (ed) *Institutional Patterns and Organizations: Culture and Environment*. Cambridge MA: Ballinger.
Douglas, M. (1986) *How Institutions Think*. New York: Syracuse University Press.
Drew, P. and Heritage, J. (1992) *Talk at Work*. Cambridge: Cambridge University Press.
Fine, G.A. (1979) Small groups and culture creation: The idioculture of little league baseball teams, *American Sociological Review*, 44, 5, 733–45.
Fligstein, N. (2001) Social skill and the theory of fields, *Sociological Theory*, 19, 2, 105–25.
Gibbs, E.P.J. (2005) Emerging zoonotic epidemics in the interconnected global community, *The Veterinary Record*, 157, 22, 673–9.
Gibbs, E.P.J. and Anderson, T.C. (2009) 'One world – one health' and the global challenge of epidemic diseases of viral aetiology, *Veterinaria Italiana*, 45, 1, 35–44.
Greger, M (2006) *Bird Flu: A Virus of Our Own Hatching*. New York: Lantern Books.
Irvine, L. (2003) The problem of unwanted pets: A case study in how institutions 'think' about clients' needs, *Social Problems*, 50, 4, 550–66.
Jones, K.E., Patel, N.G., Levy, M.A., Storeygard, A., Balk, D., Gittleman, J.L. and Daszak, P. (2008) Global trends in emerging infectious diseases, *Nature*, 451, 7181, 990–4.
Kahn, L.H. (2007) The zoonotic connection, *The Bulletin of the Atomic Scientists*, 63, 2, 68.
Kahn, K.H., Kaplan, B. and Steele, J. (2007) Confronting zoonoses through closer collaboration between medicine and veterinary medicine (as 'one medicine'), *Veterinaria Italiana*, 43, 1, 5–19.
King, L.J. (2008) Executive summary of the AVMA one health initiative task force report, *JAVMA*, 233, 2, 259–61.
Latour, B. (1988) *The Pasteurization of France*. Cambridge MA: Harvard University Press.

Lawrence, T.B. and Suddaby, R. (2006) Institutions and institutional work. In Clegg, S.R., Hardy, C., Lawrence, T. and Nord, W.R. (eds.) *The Sage Handbook of Organization Studies*. London: Sage Publications.

Leslie, M.J. and McQuiston, J.H. (2007) Surveillance for zoonotic diseases. In M'ikanatha, N., Lynfield, R., Van Beneden, C.A. and de Valk, H. (eds) *Infectious Disease Surveillance*. New York: Wiley-Blackwell.

McNeil Jr., D.G. (2004) Experts call wild birds victims, not vectors, *New York Times*, 12 October, p. F6.

McNeil Jr., D.G. (2009) No side effects so far in trial of swine flu shot, *New York Times*, 22 August, p. A10.

Morse, S.S. (2007) Global infectious disease surveillance and health intelligence, *Health Affairs*, 26, 4, 1069–77.

Rock, M., Buntain, B.J., Hatfield, J.M. and Hallgrimsson, B. (2009) Animal-human connections, 'one health', and the syndemic approach to prevention, *Social Science and Medicine*, 68, 6, 1–5.

Seidler, J. (1974) On using informants: A technique for collecting quantitative data and controlling measurement error in organizational analysis, *American Sociological Review*, 39, 6, 816–31.

Slovic, P. (1987) The Perception of Risk, *Science*, 236, 4799, 280–5.

Vaughan, D. (1996) *The Challenger Launch Decision*. Chicago IL: University of Chicago Press.

Waltner-Toews, D. (2007) *The Chickens Fight Back*. Vancouver: Greystone Books.

5

How did international agencies perceive the avian influenza problem? The adoption and manufacture of the 'One World, One Health' framework
Yu-Ju Chien

The emergence of 'One World One Health'

Since late 2003 worldwide outbreaks of highly pathogenic avian influenza (HPAI) in poultry have attracted global concerns over a possible pandemic. Scientists warned that the avian flu virus posed great pandemic threats because it might evolve into a new viral type capable of human-to-human transmission. Many inter-governmental organisations rushed to develop control and prevention policies against H5N1 avian influenza. Three international agencies are most closely associated with the tracking and control of avian flu, the World Health Organization (WHO), the Food and Agriculture Organization (FAO), and the World Organization for Animal Health (OIE). As a disease that infects both animals and humans, HPAI has challenged pre-existing specialised international governance institutions and professions.

The distinct mandated responsibilities, interests and perspectives of these international agencies soon resulted in inter-agency conflicts and tensions. The WHO, FAO and OIE are responsible for public health, food safety and animal health, respectively. They tended to govern specific domains and seldom share jurisdiction. Contradictions regarding policy prioritisation immediately appeared. For example, the WHO prioritised the necessity to strengthen pandemic preparedness for a potential outbreak, while the OIE and FAO were more concerned with eradicating viruses in poultry, a problem they considered to be imminent. FAO official Phil Harris, for example, stated that 'it is clear that avian influenza remains a *potential* risk to humans but a *real* risk to animals' (emphasis in the original).[1] In addition, tensions often escalated due to the divergent professional expertise of these agencies. For instance, public health experts at WHO and agricultural economists at FAO and OIE disagreed on large-scale culling of potentially infected birds. While WHO encouraged this strategy to avoid human infection, FAO and OIE became less willing to do so due to its impact on the food system and market. OIE's Director-General, Dr Vallat, challenged WHO's position by stating:

> Let us not forget that the WHO defines human health as not merely the absence of disease or infirmity but a state of complete physical, mental and social well-being.

Pandemics and Emerging Infectious Diseases: The Sociological Agenda, First Edition. Edited by Robert Dingwall, Lily M. Hoffman and Karen Staniland. Chapters © 2013 The Authors. Book Compilation © 2013 Foundation for the Sociology of Health & Illness / John Wiley & Sons Ltd.

Thousands of farmers, firms and employees in the poultry industry all over the world are going to disappear pointlessly. Who is going to compensate them for their distress? How long before we can say 'never again'? (Vallat 2005)

Despite tensions and disagreements, international agencies frequently expressed the need for global collaboration. The WHO, FAO and OIE developed a few collaborative platforms, such as the Global early warning system for major animal diseases, including zoonoses (GLEWS), the OIE/FAO Network of expertise on avian influenza (OFFLU),[2] and the FAO/OIE Crisis management centre for animal health (CMC-AH). In late 2008 a significant policy shift took place, when WHO, FAO and OIE, along with the United Nations Children's Fund (UNICEF), United Nations System Influenza Coordination (UNSIC), and the World Bank, jointly endorsed a 'One World, One Health' (OWOH) policy framework. Taking this concept from the Wildlife Conservation Society (WCS),[3] these agencies (re)defined OWOH as a cross-sectoral and interdisciplinary approach that recognises risks at human-animal-ecosystems interfaces. OWOH, later officially called 'One Health,' has now become a shared guiding principle for global disease prevention and control. Since then, the WHO, FAO and OIE have held and supported numerous meetings, conferences and training sessions to contemplate and promote One Health. As a European Commission officer Alain Vandermissen stated at the first One Health Congress in Melbourne, Australia, in 2011, 'One Health is now more infectious than the disease' (avian influenza).

Many experts and international officials regarded the adoption of OWOH as unprecedented and paradigm-shifting in global governance, since it demonstrated the commitment for closer organisational collaboration. In their tripartite concept note, the three agencies state that they 'realize that managing and responding to risks related to zoonoses and some high impact diseases is complex and requires multi-sectoral and multi-institutional cooperation' (FAO, OIE and WHO 2010a). However, OWOH was not clearly conceptualised when it was adopted and it is still evolving. A series of conferences and meetings have been subsequently organised to elucidate its implementation. This chapter attempts to explain why the WHO, FAO and OIE settled on and advocated OWOH, despite its vagueness. It traces the evolution of global avian flu policies to clarify the emergence, consolidation and shared appreciation of this policy frame. I argue that this global policy shift cannot be understood without examining the role of key organisational actors, who actively manufactured a new frame that reduced their conflicts and strengthened their legitimacy in a complex globalised world.

Theoretical backgrounds and methods

My research draws from and contributes to the literature on international bureaucracy, global governance, the sociology of knowledge and science and technology studies (STS). I take a constructivist approach, considering that knowledge and scientific facts are socially constructed. Gaining insights from organisational research, I focus on the roles of international agencies that connect, mobilise, empower or marginalise actors and stakeholders in crafting global norms, knowledge and policies. Scholarship that explains the formation of global models often centres upon distinct actors or forces, such as states, interest groups, civil society groups and epistemic experts. For example, the realist international relations literature considers nation-states to be the main actors in international politics; neoinstitutionalism emphasises the cultural diffusion of science and modernisation; the neoliberal school of thought highlights the overwhelming force of an increasingly integrated global market and the epistemic community theory and STS scholars focus on the networks and/or conflicts among scientists. These theories tend to treat international organisations as passive actors or simply forums. I diverge from this theoretical tendency by recognising the relative autonomy of international agencies in crafting global policies (see Barnett and Finnemore 2004, Goldman 2005).

I incorporate the international bureaucracy literature with these other lines of scholarship, revealing how international agencies actively mediate the actions and interactions of other agencies, states, experts and further stakeholders to construct knowledge of disease and global policies. This chapter argues that the OWOH policy frame gained its prominence mostly due to the increasing interaction among international agencies in a globalised world. They are key actors who constantly seek to secure their own resources, establish their legitimacy, deploy technical scientific and technological expertise and craft global responses and norms.

Specifically, by showing the conflicts, debates, and coordination among the WHO, FAO and OIE, this chapter demonstrates that the agencies are relatively autonomous actors with their own logic, interests and practices. On the one hand they have striven to reduce tensions between themselves. On the other, by advocating new policy frameworks, they have affected and reshaped the interests and behaviour of other external actors. This research illustrates the dynamic relationships between the international agencies and other global actors. It provides an important alternative organisational perspective to more structural, political economic and epistemic analyses of global policy formation and change.

In the following sections I first elucidate how the agencies utilised three competing policy frames in the early stage between 2003 and 2008, and how an OWOH framework blended these three frames to create a functional consensus. Further, I explain how officials of these agencies perceived the change and the potential and limits of the new policy frame. The findings reported here are primarily based on an analysis of policy documents from these three agencies and interviews with 34 officials at these agencies, conducted between 2008 and mid 2010.[4] Documents include updates on the disease situation, technical guidelines, standards, recommendations, reports of organisational activities and meeting minutes. The interview questions inquired into officials' responsibilities, opinions and experiences during policymaking for avian flu control.

Competition between the fragmented frames: 2003–2008

Between 2003 and 2008 the WHO, FAO and OIE drew from three competing frames to prescribe the solutions for avian flu outbreaks – the technical/biomedical intervention, a societal intervention and ecological conservation frames. These three fragmented frames, as I will call them, are often proposed and supported by distinct types of professionals. I identified these frames through document analysis and interviews based on the epidemiological assumptions and proposed control strategies entailed in policy arguments (see Table 1).

Technical/biomedical intervention frame

The first frame, a technical/biomedical intervention frame, saliently dominated the policy deliberations of these agencies in the early stage. Its rationality is deeply rooted in science and technical progress. Experts in virology, microbiology and veterinarian epidemiology and medicine constituted this frame's knowledge foundation. They assume that modern science, technologies and pharmaceuticals are the basis for disease control and prevention.

Table 1 *Four policy frames*

	Fragmented frames			
	Biomedical/ technical Frame	*Societal frame*	*Ecological conservation frame*	*One World One Health*
Norms	Modernity Development	Equality Empowerment	Environmentalism Sustainability	Modernity Equality Environmentalism
Knowledge	Virus behaviour Artefacts (antivirals, vaccines)	Human behaviour and cultures	Ecosystem Disease ecology	Interface of animal, human and ecosystems

Using this frame, international agencies often portrayed H5N1 viruses as invisible and ever-changing entities that threaten global health and security. They therefore prioritised studies on the pathogen's features, such as its molecular or genomic compositions, its infection and replication mechanisms and the development of efficient vaccines and antiviral drugs. The frame also assumes unidirectional disease transmission, in which viruses infect wild birds and wild birds transmit the viruses to poultry, through which the viruses reach humans. Proposed strategies aim at either eradicating the virus directly or impeding its transmission by applying modern medicines.

Initially, the technical/biomedical frame prevailed in global policy deliberations. The WHO, FAO and OIE advocated dissimilar technical interventions supported by each agency's specific technical expertise. For example, the FAO and OIE recommended biosecurity measures in poultry farms and markets. They urged farmers to build fences, disinfect poultry premises, adopt centralised slaughter of the birds and avoid unhygienic practices to prevent the spread of the viruses. The WHO also encouraged pharmaceutical development and stockpiling of drugs, in line with its public health expertise. This technical/biomedical frame is fundamentally expert-dominated, because only experts, particularly those with biomedical expertise, can fill current knowledge gaps and develop a magic bullet to defeat the viruses. Overall, the WHO, FAO and OIE's strategies have centred on fighting the pathogen, and their initial consensus was to 'Find it fast – kill it quickly – stop it spreading' (FAO 2008: 13).

Societal intervention frame

Although they shared the technical/biomedical frame, the three agencies still experienced great conflict when they competed for limited funding resources. Dissatisfied with the dominance of WHO's pandemic preparedness campaign, the FAO and OIE claimed that it was more efficient to control the disease at the animal source. Around 2004 and 2005 these two agencies also began to utilise a different frame – the societal intervention frame – to legitimise the agencies' significance and to distinguish themselves from the WHO.

The societal intervention frame, mostly advocated by economists and social scientists, highlights how social and cultural factors complicate disease transmission and the implementation of control strategies. Instead of exclusively focusing on the pathogen, it emphasises the need for changing human activities. Humans, in this frame, are not merely passive victims of H5N1 viruses but social actors influenced by broader structures, such as economic conditions, social trends and cultural beliefs and practices.

The societal intervention frame highlights how human activities affect disease transmission or the effectiveness of interventions. For example, some experts argued that the women and children who are often responsible for raising poultry may be at higher risk; legal or illegal trade of birds and bird products may facilitate virus transmission and certain husbandry practices such as backyard farming or intensive farming may cause threats. This frame thus recommends tailoring control strategies to particular cultures or societies. Diverse diagnostic explanations and control strategies co-exist in this model due to the diversity of socioeconomic conditions around the world. While some intervention strategies are less radical, such as promoting health education and compensating farmers for their loss, some are more radical, such as condemning and banning modern factory farming. Generally, the frame advocates more bottom-up strategies and promotes community-based programmes.

FAO and OIE's advocacy of the societal frame could be seen as an organisational strategy to enhance their political legitimacy. Firstly, by increasingly emphasising poverty alleviation, they challenged WHO's insistence on stamping out the disease by killing poultry and legitimised their policy stances. The two agencies argued that economic concerns resulted in farmers' reluctance to report suspicious outbreaks. They also noted that the mass culling of poultry often results in the poor losing their main cheap source of protein. Bringing in the societal frame therefore strengthened the FAO and OIE's legitimacy in seeking to address the problem at the agricultural level. Since 2005 the FAO and OIE have started to recommend compensating farmers to encourage disease reporting and the acceptance of culling. The FAO further proposed pro-poor risk reduction strategies to protect and enhance smallholders' livelihoods in developing countries.

Ecological conservation frame

A third frame, proposed mostly by ecological biologists, conservationists and ornithologists, focuses on wildlife and ecosystem protection. This frame emerged in 2005, when the role of wild birds in disease transmission became increasingly controversial after an outbreak in China's remote Qinghai Lake. No scientific research has yet drawn convincing conclusions on whether wild birds carry HPAI viruses during long-distance migration, due to the difficulties of large-scale wildlife surveillance research. Despite this scientific uncertainty, this frame argues that the emergence and spread of infectious diseases was mostly due to ecosystem degradation. The frame is thus more sympathetic to wild birds, compared with the other two frames. While the technical/biomedical frame assumes that wild birds are dangerous vectors that spread viruses to poultry and humans, advocates of this frame suggest that wild birds might be victims of outbreaks from intensive poultry farms.

Specifically, some wildlife experts criticised the global policy priority that has been given to short-term technical strategies, 'namely on fixing the problem rather than preventing the factors that first led to its emergence' (Rapport *et al.* 2006: 2–3). For example, a report published by the United Nations Environmental Programme identifies ecosystem degradation and ecological imbalance as root causes of emerging diseases (Rapport *et al.* 2006). This frame argues that some farming practices may exacerbate disease spread, such as the crowded conditions of factory farms, waste run off from farms to wetlands where migratory birds gather and the inadequate use of antiviral drugs that drives the mutation of influenza viruses. Proposed strategies thus seek to protect ecosystem health and wild birds.

The FAO and OIE soon responded to criticisms from wildlife experts by adopting this ecological conservation frame. They periodically and increasingly stated the necessity for investigating the role of wild birds in disease transmission. For example, one FAO's press release states:

FAO has been calling for such research [on wild birds] since early 2004, but insufficient resources have been allocated to be able to study the question properly . . . As an international agency which has invested considerable resources in numerous aspects of biodiversity preservation and conservation, FAO would be the last to pinpoint wildlife as the sole source of virus dissemination. (FAO 2006)

FAO and OIE thus organised an international scientific conference on avian influenza and wild birds to review the latest scientific knowledge in 2006. In addition, the FAO initiated a working group to address wildlife disease surveillance. Evidently, the ecological conservation frame strengthened these two agencies' legitimacy in advocating policies that represented their priorities, interests and technical expertise. They promoted interventions that required the specific veterinary expertise they were qualified to offer.

Between 2003 and 2008 the WHO, FAO and OIE often picked up different pieces of arguments from the three frames depending on the occasion. Among the three agencies, the WHO has tended to favour one-size-fits-all biomedical interventions, while FAO's policy arguments and programmes have been more diverse and fractured. The variety of FAO's arguments may be due to the relatively broad composition of its bureaucratic expertise. In addition to veterinarians, the FAO's avian flu working group also consisted of a few social scientists, communication experts and wildlife experts because of the agency's concern with food production chains. Dissimilar underlying assumptions made the FAO, OIE and WHO seem incoherent, sometimes even contradicting themselves. Tensions between these agencies clearly demonstrated their competition and conflicts. Generally, the societal and ecological conservation frames have been more peripheral than the technical/biomedical frame.

The convergence on the OWOH policy framework: 2008 to the present

Experiencing inter-agency conflicts, the WHO, FAO and OIE gradually recognised that divisions and tensions jeopardised global health governance and the organisations' legitimacy. The WHO, FAO and OIE began to recognise that the lack of cooperation between the sectors hampered cross-species disease surveillance and efficient global responses. In 2005 they started to initiate collaboration and reduce antagonisms. Specifically, cross-agency coordination first commenced to strengthen disease surveillance by sharing information on outbreaks among agencies. The WHO, FAO and OIE established working relationships through the GLEWS, OFFLU, and CMC-AH. The GLEWS, for example, tracks potential pandemic threats by exchanging outbreak information, and the OFFLU promotes the exchange of scientific information and biological materials among scientists. The three agencies also began to organise joint technical meetings and the international ministerial conferences on avian and pandemic influenza. They acknowledged that physicians, veterinarians and other health and environmental professionals should work more closely with each other to strengthen the knowledge foundation for global health governance.

The OWOH slogan, first coined by the WCS in 2004, initially did not receive much political attention. During the fifth International Ministerial Conference on Avian and Pandemic Influenza in 2007, the conference background paper, 'the New Delhi Road Map', highlighted the need for convergence between the animal health and public health sectors. The OWOH principle was recognised, and participating national delegates requested that these international agencies prepare a strategic frame to guide country responses. The FAO, WHO, OIE, UNICEF, UNSIC and the World Bank thus jointly produced and endorsed the 'Contributing to "One World, One Health" strategic framework' during the following

International Ministerial Conference on Avian and Pandemic Influenza in 2008. This document was exclusively drafted and discussed among six officials from these six agencies, without consulting external experts. It laid out five main strategies[5] geared to reducing risk at the animal-human-ecosystems interfaces. Specifically, the framework highlights a cross-sectoral and multidisciplinary approach that recognises the intricate relationships between human, animal and ecosystem health. After this conference, the OWOH policy framework became the guiding principle for global health governance, which proposes that managing novel pathogens requires collaboration between different professions and international agencies.

In principle, OWOH is a frame that seeks to combine the three competing fragmented frames discussed above, acknowledging that various multiple factors all contribute to disease transmission. It also seems to merge all values emphasised by the three fragmented frames, including modernity, social empowerment and sustainability. Seemingly holistic, the frame was primarily conceptual and not clearly defined when it was released. Most officials at the three agencies recognised that the OWOH slogan is catchy and appropriate. However, until 2009, when I interviewed most officials, they could not articulate its meaning and practical steps. To most of them, OWOH is more of an abstract concept than a set of concrete policies.

To translate this abstract framework into action, the WHO, FAO and OIE subsequently organised several consultation and technical meetings. For example, in 2009 the Public Health Agency of Canada hosted a consultation meeting in Winnipeg. In May 2010 the Centers for Disease Control and Prevention in the US hosted another consultation meeting to operationalise the concept. In February 2011 Australia's Commonwealth Scientific and Industrial Research Organisation hosted the first One Health Congress to showcase relevant research and policy implementation. In 2011 the Mexican government hosted another high level technical meeting to address health risks at human-animal-ecosystems interfaces. The participants of these meetings were mostly invited international experts with medical or veterinarian backgrounds, officials of international agencies and national delegates from both the public health and agricultural sectors. Since 2008 the three agencies have frequently expressed their enthusiasm for OWOH. In 2010 the WHO, FAO and OIE (2010a) jointly published a 'Tripartite concept note' to reiterate their commitment to inter-agency collaboration. They also changed OWOH to 'One Health' to recognise the WCS' possession of the original phrase.

In the meetings to conceptualise One Health, nonetheless, participants struggled to give it a clear definition. After an FAO-OIE-WHO joint technical consultation in 2008, meeting participants agreed that 'it became clear that this concept [One Health] was not new; however, the roles and strategies of all the players globally are not fully understood nor effectively integrated' (FAO, OIE and WHO 2010b: 13). Some meetings ended with a conclusion that clear definitions and consistency of One Health are necessary. Most of the time, the scope of OWOH was left open or carried to the next appropriate meeting. One OIE officer summarised what she observed at the Winnipeg 2009 meeting:

> For some people [at the meeting], this [OWOH] means to investigate the animal-and-human interface, while others believed that food security is more important. Still other experts thought that health issues should be more broadly defined, including not only disease prevention but also healthy life styles. The final consensus of the meeting was that One World, One Health could mean whatever people want to. Each country can emphasise any aspect relevant to the animal-human-ecosystem interfaces. (09–2009, interview)

This vagueness of One Health persists. Two years later, during the first One Health Congress in early 2011, experts and public officials still struggled to come up with a consensual definition. For example, in the opening plenary speech, one senior FAO official commented:

> One Health means different things to different people. If you ask 10 people here, you may get 10 different ideas. We may not eventually obtain an agreement on One Health in this room. However, all of us believe that it is important . . . During the next three days, we will discuss and conceptualise One Health in order to put our words to practice. (Field notes, 2011)

Experts participating in the congress continued to debate the scope and definition of One Health. Some insisted on focusing on infectious diseases, while others believed that One Health should include promoting healthy lifestyles and securing nutrients. Several participants and speakers recognised that having a clear definition of One Health was difficult and that stakeholders were still free to prioritise tasks differently.

Interestingly, despite One Health's vagueness, policymakers, experts, and international agencies all welcomed the concept. The endorsement of One Health clearly did not result from a solid scientific understanding of the complex epidemiological dynamics – international agencies and experts repeatedly acknowledged the existing knowledge gaps in disease transmission mechanisms. Neither could the policy shift be entirely attributed to international politics, because most powerful nation–states and donors were more interested in efficiently preventing diseases from threatening the West by containing them.

The endorsement of OWOH, I argue, was mostly driven by the tensions and growing interactions between specialised international agencies in an increasingly globalised world that challenged the legitimacy of specialised governance institutions. It became a step toward appeasing cross-agency contradictions and forging consensus among them and with other global actors, such as divided professionals, self-interested nation–states and development-oriented donors. By merging different normative claims, knowledge foundations and policies from fragmented frames, the WHO, FAO and OIE attempted to reduce cross-agency conflicts, avoid criticisms and create a global consensus that facilitated coordination.

Functional consensus despite diverse interpretations

The political function of OWOH was illustrated by officials' diverse and sometimes contradictory interpretations of this concept. My interviews disclosed three distinct perspectives regarding OWOH: those who bought into the idea, others who were content with current technical cooperation and yet others who considered OWOH a strategic response. Yet international officials all welcomed One Health no matter what perspective they held.

First, some officials wholeheartedly embraced One Health, praising it as a momentous paradigm shift in global governance. For instance, a WHO official commented that OWOH was 'a new perspective that international organisations embrace'. She elaborated, 'We've learned the importance of cooperation over the years' (W10–2008, interview). Another FAO official said:

> One Health is to broaden the veterinary approach. In the past, you wait for the disease to emerge; you respond to it, you get rid of it. In One Health, you try to understand the factors that lead diseases to emerge. You try to broaden the spectrum

of professionals: use communication specialists, socio-economists, bring doctors and vets together. (F9–2010, interview)

These officials were enthusiastic about capturing a big picture of disease epidemiology.

Other officials believed that OWOH just consolidated ongoing inter-agency cooperation in global disease surveillance. One WHO official commented, 'Some people consider OWOH a new idea, but actually we have being doing this for a long time. We just didn't use this phrase' (W8–2009, interview). He, along with other officials, considered that One Health was a reaffirmation of their ongoing technical collaboration rather than a paradigm shift. Another WHO officer held a similar opinion, arguing that OWOH just crystallised what had already happened:

It gives it a name. An expectation of a name seems to make sense. It helps us to capitalise what we have achieved and show that we can do more . . . It's just a concept, a vision. Hopefully it will underline the work we do.

This interviewee continued, 'I don't want to see a new programme that diverts the attention to the animal and human interface, because it's already been there' (W7–2009, interview). Some argue that the principle only 'put what the organisations had been doing in words' (W10–2009, interview).

Lastly, several officials considered OWOH beneficial for sustaining donors' interests and investments in avian flu. For them, the adoption of OWOH was, at least partially, a strategic move. It was advocated primarily for reigniting global attention to avian flu prevention and control. During my fieldwork in 2009, several officials expressed an anxiety about 'avian flu fatigue,' that is, fading global attention to avian flu because the expected pandemic had not occurred. To them, the OWOH frame helped refocus global attention, particularly the financial commitment of donors such as the European Commission, the United States Agency for International Development and the World Bank. Many officials noted, 'We have to let the funding agencies understand that the investment is beneficial' (F9–2010). Another WHO official added, 'Each organisation has its own agenda. We find the collaboration beneficial. But we need political support to make it happen' (W6–2008, interview). Another consultant similarly commented that One Health is a:

repackaging of what has been happening for the past 30 years to make it more attractive to donors – there is a need for cross-disciplinary coordination, but it has always been this way. (E17–2010, survey response)

Noticeably, no matter how these bureaucrats interpreted One Health, they recognised its significance. The three agencies also attempted to redefine the meanings and strategies of One Health by initiating discussions among international agencies, experts, and donors through organised meetings and conferences. Their shared enthusiasm but dissimilar interpretations of One Health illustrate the framework's function as a boundary object strategically used by the WHO, FAO and OIE to transform tensions and encourage coordination (Star and Griesemer 1989).

Star and Griesemer (1989) state that a boundary object is 'plastic enough to adapt to local needs and the constraints of the several parties employing them, yet robust enough to maintain a common identity across sites' (1989: 393). One Health comprises characteristics of a boundary object for being both robust and flexible. On one hand, specialised organisational actors and experts supported One Health due to their common objective in promoting heath. By recognising that human, animal and ecosystem health are intertwined, One Health legitimised participation by all agencies in knowledge and policy construction. On the other hand, One Health also allows dissimilar interpretations, as it includes all the essentials of fragmented frames, recognises every possible epidemiological factor, and affirms different values. As an all-you-can-eat type of framework, OWOH allows users to identify with different pieces of the frame. The 'productive vagueness' of One Health as a result facilitates communication among previously independent social worlds.

Consequently, OWOH created a sense of harmony across agencies and stakeholders with dissimilar interests and focuses. They may not necessarily interpret and implement OWOH in the same way, yet they now share a common vision and a commitment to 'get along' (Halfon 2006). Under the big umbrella of OWOH, individual bureaucrats, organisations, and experts downplay their conflicts and competition and reach the consensus that they are in fact complementary. Disputes over prioritisation were somewhat alleviated, as they no longer needed to choose one over another. Their growing collaboration also established the collective legitimacy of the three agencies.

A double-edged policy framework

The evolution of OWOH in response to avian flu outbreaks demonstrates the influence of international agencies on global policymaking and policy change. The globalisation of pathogens has not only penetrated national boundaries, but it also challenged existing specialised bureaucratic governance systems and professionalised production of disease knowledge. The political endorsement of One Health was not simply driven by the advance of science, politics between influential nations and stakeholders, or advocacy networks of experts. Rather, competition and coordination between the WHO, FAO and OIE essentially shaped and promoted this new global health governance regime, which has now gone beyond avian flu and extended to other infectious diseases and pandemic threats. Ongoing institutional promotion and articulation of One Health illustrates that international agencies, though limited by their mandates and technical expertise, are not static. They can proactively respond to challenges, conflicts, and criticisms by adjusting policy claims and frames.

This research therefore contributes to the international bureaucracy literature by showing how world organisations shape disease knowledge and political policies by interacting, mobilising and networking with other global actors. The WHO, FAO and OIE strategically borrowed the concept OWOH from the WCS, transformed it into an overarching political principle, and consistently reconstructed its meanings and implementations. The emergence and popularity of OWOH can be attributed to negotiations and compromises between these principal organisational actors. It became appealing and widely appreciated before a clear definition and agreement on practical strategies was achieved. By adopting OWOH, the WHO, FAO and OIE not only reduced tensions among themselves and advanced their own legitimacy, but they also reshaped the institutional environment and interests of other stakeholders. For instance, these agencies began to encourage scientific investigations on the complexity at the animal-human-ecosystem interfaces. They advocated for multi-disciplinary collaboration between medical, veterinary, wildlife and other professionals. The WHO, FAO and OIE also began to cultivate expert networks of One Health through organised consultation and technical meetings. Some experts and public officials have now identified themselves as One Health advocates and practitioners. In addition, these agencies sought to motivate donors and member states to continue investing in disease control and pandemic preparedness. Several officials emphasised the importance of 'educating' donors and of encouraging nation states to promote One Health. As one FAO official commented, 'It is very important to convince donors to support OWOH. Because donors are like politicians, they are usually more interested in emergency responses rather than long-term programmes' (F4–2010, interview).

Moreover, this research complements the neo-institutional approach by illustrating how new global norms and models come about. Neo-institutionalism elucidates how broader cultural beliefs structure organisational cognition and guide decision-making (Schofer *et al.* 2012). However, how these norms and rules emerge and how they become crystallised has not been adequately explained. Neither has much work explored how organisations respond to multiple, and sometimes competing, logics. This study shows that integration and abstraction could be one organisational strategy in response to norm contradictions. The WHO, FAO and OIE have shrewdly merged dissimilar values and knowledge claims to avoid tensions and criticisms. They incorporated distinct norms, including scientific advancement, social justice and ecological sustainability, into an all-inclusive framework by means of numerous technical, consultation and political meetings. OWOH's meaning has been fluid, varying with contexts and users.

This flexibility has both potential and limits. Although OWOH provides functional consensus due to its versatility, this very characteristic could prevent fundamental cognitive and behaviour changes. Its vagueness allows different, or even conflicting, interpretations and strategies to coexist. Yet, without shared concrete strategies except consensus on the need for collaboration, it could be little more than ceremonial. The earlier interventions of the WHO, FAO, and OIE have been criticised for advocating top-down and technocratic approaches (Scoones and Forster 2008), for ignoring key factors of disease transmission such as intensive commercial farming (Davis 2005, Wallace 2009) and for representing certain farming practices as backward or problematic (Bingham and Hinchliffe 2008).

Although OWOH incorporates the fragmented frames, it does not always promise policy changes. For example, officials and experts who accept the technical/biomedical frame can embrace OWOH without shifting their perspectives. Rather, OWOH may downplay tensions and essential differences between frames. Most international officials have quickly learned to speak and apply the new pattern of reasoning by developing optimistic statements and abstract blueprints. If officials perceive One Health only as a strategy to avoid tensions or to refocus political attention, they can still practise the dominant technical/biomedical frame without converting to the seemingly holistic One Health perspective.

Officials, in addition, tend to resist change. During my interviews in 2009 and early 2010, some officials recognised that the political endorsement of OWOH had not considerably changed their work despite the fact that cross-agency technical cooperative programmes had already been established. Several officials confirmed that 'We are doing the same work, whether we have this phrase OWOH or not' (F14–2010, interview). Another WHO official insisted that OWOH is only a concept. He said

Don't think that it [OWOH] is something that's too concrete. It's a new concept. We are not aiming at producing new programmes . . . There are partnerships to advocate the new concept, to use the concept. But those are partnerships, not new programmes. (W8–2009, interview)

These officials' perception of the continuity of previous work suggests that international agencies tend to maintain their governance territories and resist the changes in bureaucratic structures that One Health demands.

In the age of globalisation, a framework like OWOH with a more sophisticated understanding of disease causality and management is certainly welcomed by many actors. Undoubtedly, improved cross-sectoral surveillance platforms such as the GLEWS have facilitated quick detection and contingency responses to disease outbreaks. Despite these improvements in technical cooperation and strategies, whether the WHO, FAO and OIE will overcome barriers of bureaucratic divisions, professional specialisation, and international politics to realise One Health is still up in the air. The evolution of One Health, nevertheless, demonstrates that global problems and solutions are products of policy negotiations, in which international agencies can mediate and direct global policy formation and change. Motivated by resource interests and a desire for legitimacy, they have not only shaped knowledge of infectious diseases but also constructed policy responses to associated pandemic threats.

Acknowledgements

The author thanks Joachim J. Savelsberg, Elizabeth H. Boyle, Sarah Barker and anonymous reviewers for valuable advice. Research funding was provided by the Social Science Research Council; and the University of Minnesota Consortium on Law and Values in Health, Environment & the Life Sciences, Office of International Programs, Graduate School, Center for German and European Studies, and Department of Sociology.

Notes

1   Harris (2006) was an information officer of FAO's Emergency Centre for Transboundary Animal Diseases.
2   OFFLU was renamed the OIE/FAO Network of Expertise on Animal Influenza after the H1N1 influenza pandemic in 2009.
3   'One World One Health' was also called the 12 Manhattan Principles. Its primary goal was to prevent epidemic and epizootic disease and to maintain ecosystem integrity holistically (Wildlife Conservation Society n.d.).
4   I focus on the WHO, FAO and OIE while leaving out the UNSIC, UNCEF and World Bank because the former agencies are considered as having technical expertise on avian influenza. Due to institutional review board requirements, I have maintained the confidentiality of my informants. Interview quotes are thus presented by their code numbers.
5   The five strategies in the OWOH policy framework include: (i) building robust public and animal health systems that comply with the WHO's international health regulations and OIE standards, (ii) preventing and controlling disease outbreaks by improving national and international response capacities, (iii) addressing the needs of poor populations by shifting focuses to developing economies and locally important diseases, (iv) promoting collaboration across sectors and disciplines and (v) conducting research that guides the development of targeted disease control programmes.

References

Barnett, M.N. and Finnemore, M. (2004) *Rules for the World: International Organizations in Global Politics*. Ithaca: Cornell University Press.
Bingham, N. and Hinchliffe, S. (2008) Mapping the multiplicities of biosecurity. In Lakoff, A. and Collier, S.J. (eds) *Biosecurity Interventions*. New York: Columbia University Press.

Davis, M. (2005) *The Monster at Our Door: The Global Threat of Avian Flu*. New York: New Press.

Food and Agriculture Organization (FAO) (2006) Avian flu: don't place all the blame on wild birds. Available at http://www.fao.org/docs/eims/upload/214442/Dontplaceallblameonwildbirds.pdf (accessed 5 September 2012).

FAO (2008) *Biosecurity for highly pathogenic avian influenza: issues and options*. Rome. Available at ftp://ftp.fao.org/docrep/fao/011/i0359e/i0359e00.pdf (accessed 5 September 2012).

FAO, World Organization for Animal Health (OIE) and World Health Organization (WHO) (2010a) The FAO-OIE-WHO Collaboration: sharing responsibilities and coordinating global activities to address health risks at the animal-human-ecosystems interfaces. A tripartite concept note. Available at http:// www.fao.org/docrep/012/ak736e/ak736e00.pdf (accessed 5 September 2012).

FAO, OIE and WHO (2010b) FAO-OIE-WHO joint technical consultation on avian influenza at the human–animal interface, *Influenza and Other Respiratory Viruses*, 4, Suppl. 1, 1–29.

Goldman, M. (2005) *Imperial Nature: The World Bank and Struggles for Social Justice in the Age of Globalization*. New Haven and London: Yale University Press.

Halfon, S. (2006) The disunity of consensus: international population policy coordination as socio-technical practice, *Social Studies of Science*, 36, 5, 783–807.

Harris, P. (2006) Avian influenza: an animal health issue. Available at http://www.fao.org/avianflu/en/issue.html (accessed 5 September 2012).

Rapport, D.J., Howard, J., Maffi, L. and Mitchell, B. (2006) Avian influenza and the environment: an ecohealth perspective. *A Report Submitted to UNEP. EcoHealth Consulting*. New York: UNEP.

Schofer, E. Hironaka, A. Frank, D.J. and Longhofer, W. (2012) Sociological institutionalism and world society. In Amenta E., Nash, K. and Scott A. (eds) *The Wiley-Blackwell Companion to Political Sociology*. New York: Wiley-Blackwell.

Scoones, I. and Forster, P. (2008) *The international response to highly pathogenic avian influenza: science, policy, and politics*. STEPS Working Paper 10. Brighton: STEPS Centre.

Star, S.L. and Griesemer, J.R. (1989) Institutional ecology, 'translations' and boundary objects: amateurs and professionals in Berkeley's museum of vertebrate zoology, 1907–39, *Social Studies of Science*, 19, 3, 387–420.

Vallat, B. (2005) A big thank-you to the Geneva Meeting. Available at http://www.oie.int/for-the-media/editorials/detail/article/a-big-thank-you-to-the-geneva-meeting/ (accessed 5 September 2012).

Wallace, R.G. (2009) Breeding influenza: the political virology of offshore farming, *Antipode*, 41, 5, 916–51.

Wildlife Conservation Society (n.d.) One World One Health. Available at http://www.wcs.org/conservation-challenges/wildlife-health/wildlife-humans-and-livestock/one-world-one-health.aspx (accessed 5 September 2012).

6

Global health risks and cosmopolitisation: from emergence to interference

Muriel Figuié

Introduction

International health organisations and western nations are exerting growing pressure on other countries to cooperate in managing health risks such as emerging diseases, as demonstrated during the recent episodes of severe acute respiratory syndrome (SARS) and avian flu (Scoones 2010). This pressure is being exerted on countries with different perceptions of risks and with different agendas (Renn 2008, Taylor-Gooby and Zinn 2006). In this chapter I examine how risks defined as 'global' by stakeholders in the international community push nations toward a cosmopolitisation of their risk management policies, together with the mechanisms used and the intended and unintended outcomes. I use Beck's World at Risk theory (Beck 2009) to study one empirical case: Vietnam's management of a recent emerging disease, the highly pathogenic avian influenza (HPAI), which is associated with the avian flu virus (H5N1), and popularly known as avian flu, avian influenza or bird flu. This study covers the period from 2003 to 2007, a period of intense international activity in avian flu management. I will discuss the link between global risks and cosmopolitisation, as identified by Beck. The following sections show how avian flu has been framed by international organisations and how Vietnam has complied with this definition, under pressure from the US administration and international organisations such as the World Health Organization (WHO), the World Organization for Animal Health (OIE) and the Food and Agriculture Organization (FAO). I analyse the mechanisms of this convergence and its consequences for Vietnam. Finally, the discussion addresses the role of country reputation, national sovereignty, community of interests, community of fear and values as driving forces for a cosmopolitisation of health policy.

Materials and method

I conducted a comprehensive review of all the grey literature documents on avian flu issued by the Vietnamese ministries of health, and agriculture and rural development, of official documents on Vietnam's strategy for avian flu (known as the 'Red Book' and the 'Green Book') and regulations adopted by the Vietnamese government, as well as expert reports from international and foreign organisations (FAO, WHO, Agrifood Consulting

Pandemics and Emerging Infectious Diseases: The Sociological Agenda, First Edition. Edited by Robert Dingwall, Lily M. Hoffman and Karen Staniland. Chapters © 2013 The Authors. Book Compilation © 2013 Foundation for the Sociology of Health & Illness / John Wiley & Sons Ltd.

International and Agence Franç aise de Développement). In-depth interviews were conducted in 2007 and 2008 with key informants involved directly in Vietnamese avian flu management. In total, 20 people were interviewed, half of whom were working in public or private Vietnamese organisations (and representing the Ministry of Agriculture and Rural Development [MARD], the Ministry of Health [MOH] and the veterinary services of two provinces, as well as representatives of the private sector). The other half were stakeholders from the international community (members of the FAO avian influenza team; experts in infectious diseases working for the WHO, members of the Partnership for Avian and Human Influenza (PAHI), representatives of foreign non-governmental organisations (NGOs) active on the topic and one member of the leadership of an international hospital). Interviewees were asked to relate the role of the different stakeholders in the avian flu management over time and the major points of debates and controversies. Most interviews were conducted in English, with a few in Vietnamese through a translator. Interviewees were guaranteed anonymity. Some people have been interviewed twice or even three times. The interviews were recorded wherever possible and transcribed for further in-depth analysis. Additional information was collected from the websites of the FAO, OIE and WHO on avian flu and SARS, on the 'One World One Health' strategic framework adopted by these organisations, on the International Health Regulation of the WHO, and on the Terrestrial Animal Health Code of OIE.

Global risks and cosmopolitisation

The theory of risk society (Beck 1992) describes the transition of societies from first modernity (or industrial societies) to second modernity (or late modernity). Second modernity is characterised by global risks or, more exactly, global anticipated uncertainties. For Beck (2009) global risks (or late modern risks) are both real and constructed. On the realist side, global risks are manmade, produced by industrial modernisation and linked to globalisation. They are incalculable, since their destructive potential to health and the environment may have long-term and large-scale effects.

On the constructivist side, global risks are produced by the ambition of late modern societies to anticipate and control potential catastrophes. As anticipated catastrophes, global risks take the form of contested knowledge: 'their reality can be dramatised or minimised, transformed or simply denied according to the norms which decide what is known and what is not' (Beck 2009: 30). Consequently, late modern societies are confronted with a diversity of viewpoints and values from which risks can be evaluated. This situation creates the potential for new forms of risk governance involving a wide network of stakeholders and creating opportunities for an 'involuntary democratization' (Beck 2009: 60).

Beck's theory has been widely criticised for its Eurocentrism, even by Beck himself (Beck and Grande 2010, Dingwall 1999, Mythen 2007). In response, Beck and his associates have developed the World at Risk theory (Beck 2009, Beck and Grande 2010). They have introduced the concept of cosmopolitan modernities in order to take into account the varieties of modernity according to specific national cultures and histories and their global interdependencies. One of the main issues addressed by the World at Risk theory is: how do countries on different paths towards modernity, and with different risk perceptions, cooperate or not, in order to confront shared global risks? This question emphasises the realist dimension of global risk, since it opposes the diversities in risk perceptions to the nature of late modern risks. Beck has been criticised for the ambiguous status of risk in his theory.

According to Burgess (2006), in many works inspired by this theory, risks remain given, objectified and decontextualised, despite a proclaimed constructionist approach: their scientific and politically manufactured dimensions are often neglected. For Mythen (2007: 800, quoting Lash: 51), 'so far as perceptions of risk are concerned Beck leans heavily towards the realist position'.

This chapter attempts to show that the framing of a risk as a global risk (that is, according to Beck's definition, as a potential threat) varies according to stakeholders and over time. It will contextualise and exemplify Beck's assertion that:

> Global risks provide a basis of legitimation for political institutions and social movements that press for more humane forms of globalisation, which does not preclude, of course, that this cosmopolitan moment can be instrumentalised for ideological purposes. (Beck 2009: 20–1)

Avian flu: a classic and a modern risk

H5N1, the virus responsible for avian flu (more exactly, responsible for a HPAI) may be framed either as a classic risk or as a risk of second modernity. Experts of international organisations consider avian flu and emerging diseases in general as products of a globalised environment requiring global answers (FAO *et al.* 2008, OIE 2009, WHO 2007b). The virus first appeared in Hong Kong in 1997 and then re-emerged in Vietnam and China in 2003 before spreading to more than 62 other countries over the last nine years:

> Today more than ever the international spread of diseases or other risks threatens health, economies, and security. No country can 'go it alone' in protecting its citizens from the threats. (WHO 2007b: 2)

And the director of the OIE, Dr B. Vallat (2007: 1) declared: 'Indeed, a single country failing to control animal disease outbreaks could put the entire World at Risk'.

Is this characteristic enough to define avian influenza as a risk of second or late modernity? Different authors (Burgess 2006, Boudia and Jas 2007, Dingwall 1999, Méric *et al.* 2009) have criticised Beck's claim about the newness of risks of global scale and his lack of a historical perspective. But risks of second modernity are not just global risks – they are an anticipation of threat.

Avian flu poses a three-dimensional risk. Firstly, it is an epizootic disease, that is, a disease causing high mortality in an animal population; in this case poultry raised by farmers and wild birds. Secondly, it is also a zoonotic disease: it can be transmitted from poultry to humans but its impact has been limited compared to other infectious diseases (352 fatalities worldwide since 2003). But thirdly, experts fear that the virus might mutate into a form that is transmissible from human to human, which could provoke a human influenza pandemic with high mortality. This mutation could be just a question of time: as Dr Nabarro, the UN coordinator for avian flu declared in answering the question 'What is the probability of a pandemic?' to a journalist from the *Poultry Diseases* network, 2007):

> [W]e cannot say with any certainty at all when it would happen, where it would start, how severe it would be. So the only certainty we can share with each other is that it would happen one day.

In a joint press release on 27 January FAO *et al.* (2004) describe avian flu as a serious threat to humanity. Different stakeholders (such as farmers, consumers and policymakers), living on different paths of modernity with different risk cultures may focus on one dimension or another of avian flu: epizootic, zoonotic or pandemic. As an epizootic or zoonotic disease, H5N1 is a classic risk. As a pandemic threat, avian flu is a risk of second modernity, according to Beck's definition. And that is the way international organisations have framed it.

Avian flu (H5N1) marks a new stage in the internationalisation and globalisation of action to control health. First, the management of this risk by international health organisations indicates 'a colonisation of the future', in the words of Beck (2003: 29). It marks the unprecedented ambition of the institutions in charge of managing human and animal health risks to prepare the world for a virus that still does not exist but which could emerge from a mutation of H5N1. Secondly, the discourses produced by international organisations mark the end of a discourse that everything is under control. In a WHO handbook on avian flu published for journalists (WHO 2005b) one can read: 'the great unknown: why there are no certain answers for the big questions' (p. 4) as well as, throughout the text: 'we don't know' (p. 5), 'unpredictable' (p. 10), 'uncertain' (p. 10). Thirdly, H5N1 and SARS have opened the way for global health governance with an extended scope of intervention for international organisations and greater interference (see Calain 2007 for the WHO strategy). New WHO and OIE regulations encourage nations to go beyond routine measures on borders and to adopt preventive measures at the source of contamination, that is, within affected countries. Member states' obligations have been extended to the declaration of any 'extraordinary public health event which constitutes a public health risk to other States through the international spread of disease, and may require a coordinated international response' (WHO 2005c: 1). Lastly, the WHO and OIE are now authorised to take note of any information source on disease outbreaks in addition to official notifications from national administrations. Dr Chan, Director-General of WHO (2007a: xv), noted: 'This reflects a new reality in a world of instant communications: the concealment of disease outbreaks is no longer a viable option for governments'.

The framing of avian flu by international organisations (WHO, OIE, FAO) illustrates a high porosity between the spaces of international stakeholders involved in health issues and academic researchers on risk society. The new paradigm 'One World One Health' elaborated by international organisations (FAO *et al.* 2008) calls countries and actors (private, public; administration and civil society; experts of animal, human and environment health) to transcend boundaries, to progressively construct shared perceptions of health risks and to build coordinated responses to global health issues. This paradigm reflects what Beck calls a community of fate and a community of responsibility. But the current results are far from 'cosmopolitan moment' (Beck 2009: 47) in which nations see themselves as parts of a community of threat and fate and voluntarily contribute to global cooperation. According to Beck (2009: 57) global risks could open up 'a moral and political space that can give rise to a culture of responsibility that transcends borders and conflicts' but this opportunity has not been seized in the case of avian flu.

Conversely, Scoones (2010) has shown that the new global health governance is dominated by a Northern perspective that ignores the structural inequalities of access to resources and exposure to risk. Moreover it forces poor countries to focus on a potential catastrophe when they already lack the resources to address classic infectious diseases like meningitis or malaria (Calain 2007). Global risks push for a globalisation of health governance. But global risks also presuppose the existence of international organisations that manufacture uncertainties through a performative discourse justifying an extended scope of intervention for themselves.

Did the perception and framing of avian flu by international health organisations converge in Vietnam or did it reveal a clash in risk cultures? Global risks being in Beck's theory, a product, as well as a driving force of late modernisation, Vietnam's experience of modernisation needs to be described before answering this question.

Asia, Vietnam and cosmopolitan modernities

Studies have been conducted to provide Beck's risk theory with an empirical basis and to confront it with the contexts of non-western countries, including Asian countries (see Calhoun 2010 and the articles in the *British Journal of Sociology* 2010). These studies have underlined specific characteristics associated with modernisation in emerging Asiatic countries. Firstly, the rapidity of processes such as industrialisation, urbanisation and economic liberalisation, lead to the almost simultaneous development of first modernity and the transition to a second one, resulting in a compressed modernity (Beck and Grande 2010, Chang 2010, Kyung-Sup 2010). Secondly, 'global risks as a driving force of second modernity are more relevant in East Asia as a result of the side effects of the rush to development' (Han and Shim 2010: 465). Thirdly, the economic and political transition has meant 'the protracted coexistence of socialist, capitalist or even (neo) traditionalist components of the political economy, thereby imposing an ultra-complex (compressed) modernity' as shown by Kyung-Sup (2010: 457) in analysing China. These works focus on global risks as a structural, objective factor and do little to document their local framing and local perception.

The recent history of the Socialist Republic of Vietnam illustrates this rush to development and the transition towards an ultra-complex modernity. In the 1980s Vietnam was considered one of the world's poorest countries (Vietnam Development Report 2004) and was economically and politically isolated. The country is now classified as a middle income country by the International Monetary Fund and is a member of numerous international organisations and forums.

Following the establishment of the communist government in 1955, the victory over American armed forces in 1974 and the invasion of Cambodia in 1978, Vietnam suffered a US trade embargo and an international boycott. Vietnam also lost considerable support following the collapse of the Soviet Union. In the 1980s the domestic economic situation was a disaster, resulting in famines. In reaction, Vietnam implemented from 1986 important economic and political reforms (known as Doi Moi). At the international level Vietnam's objective was to become integrated in the international community. But according to Do Hien (2004: 171, my translation), at that time, 'winning back the confidence of the international community was an almost impossible challenge'. Nevertheless, Vietnam succeeded within a relatively short time. The country started by restoring its relationship with China following the end of the conflict in Cambodia (1989) and then by amplifying its relations with neighbouring South-East Asian countries. Vietnam made an important gesture when it agreed to cooperate with the USA over the 'missing in action' affair (1986). This led to the lifting of the trade embargo (1994), after which Vietnam regained access to international credit (from the Asian Development Bank and the International Monetary Fund) and was integrated into the coalition of South-East Asian countries in 1995 (Do Hien 2004). When avian flu emerged in Vietnam these successes were considered by Vietnamese authorities as steps towards a longer term objective: Vietnam's integration into the World Trade Organization.

At the national level, the liberalisation of the former planned economy has provoked unprecedented economic growth with positive outcomes such as poverty alleviation, the reduction of malnutrition and increased wealth (Vietnam Development Report 2004). The political consequences are more complex. Bao An and de Tréglodé (2004) have shown how, through these reforms and in a very pragmatic way, Vietnamese authorities combine contradictory forces: economic and social dynamics with ideological and political continuity, a project of modernisation with patriotic, historic and cultural references. According to these authors, the role of the state and the Communist Party has not been weakened by this modernisation process. The process is kept within the ruling system of a bureaucratic–authoritarian state with a single party. The state has retained its monopoly in decision-making and the party is responsible for guaranteeing the continuity of moral values throughout the economic development process. Nevertheless, the growing gap between rules and practices opens space for initiatives but without allowing the emergence of a real opposition (Bao An and de Tréglodé 2004). These characteristics of Vietnam's modernisation have affected Vietnam's cooperation with the international community to deal with avian flu.

Relations of definitions, relations of domination: the framing of avian flu

The first human casualties caused by the re-emergence of the H5N1 were officially recorded in Vietnam and China in 2003. This put Vietnam, according to international organisations such as the WHO, OIE and FAO, in the front line of the war against the virus. Vietnam currently ranks second in human deaths from H5N1 (352 deaths, WHO 2012) and numerous poultry outbreaks are still being recorded (World Organization for Animal Health [OIE] 2012).

I identify two phases in Vietnam's management of the virus. The first began with the first outbreaks of the virus in Vietnam; the second began with the arrival of the virus in Europe and the globalisation of its management.

Phase 1: avian flu, a classic risk
The first phase began at the end of 2003 and the start of 2004. It was a consequence of a local epidemic (in which up to nine cases of human contamination per month were being recorded), as well as the number of infected flocks (as many as 25 per cent of Vietnamese communes had contaminated poultry flocks). Avian flu was rapidly compared with SARS by experts and the media, who feared an explosive increase in human cases. The SARS virus had emerged in China in 2002, reaching Vietnam and going on to kill 774 people throughout the world in a few months. The daily newspaper *Thanh Nien* (2004: 1) published the following headline: 'a flu epidemic even more dangerous than SARS'.

The SARS virus is transmissible from human to human, but the mode of transmission of H5N1 to humans was then unclear. The Vietnamese authorities and the WHO had been criticised for their slow response to SARS. In the case of avian flu, Vietnamese authorities were supported by the international organisations (WHO, OIE and FAO) for a prompt answer. They took unprecedented measures: a massive culling operation of 17 per cent of all poultry in less than three months (Agrifood Consulting International [ACI] 2007), as well as the restriction of all transport of poultry across provincial and national borders:

> If there had been only avian flu, people would have thought the WHO was going mad, overreacting. But before, when we had the SARS, the WHO were criticised for not acting quickly enough. (Doctor, international medical cooperation, interview, 2 May 2008)

The Vietnamese Communist Party published decrees and actively intervened in the preventative culling operation, mobilising the army as well as the party-affiliated associations of the Patriotic Front (Guénel and Klingberg 2010, Tuong 2010). The network of actors mobilised closely resembles that which is normally seen in this country in the event of floods, typhoons or even past armed conflicts:

> The rapidity of Vietnam's response can be explained by its history. This country has had to mobilise the population on numerous occasions throughout the past. I was born in peacetime, but I am imbued with this Vietnamese culture of collective struggle. (Representative from the Ministry of Agriculture, interview, 23 May 2008)

As one expert in an international organisation noted:

> Vietnamese people are accustomed and prepared to face situations of emergency. They do not have to worry about media, public opinion, or sectoral interests . . . And they have no complexes. Moreover the chain of command, the Communist Party and the army, is very efficient. (International expert, interview, 10 December 2007)

In contrast with this initial mobilisation, avian flu lost its place on the political and media agenda a few months later. Regular outbreaks were recorded among poultry but human mortality remained low compared with the past SARS outbreak and other infectious diseases already present in Vietnam. The population's anxiety receded: consumers resumed poultry consumption after a dramatic drop (Figuié and Fournier 2008) and poultry farmers finally perceived avian flu as just another epizootic disease (Desvaux and Figuié 2011). The problem was reduced to a veterinary problem to be managed by the Ministry of Agriculture. At the same time, developed countries were adopting national protective strategies such as the production and stockpiling of vaccines and masks (Gilbert 2007).

Phase 2: avian flu, a modern risk
In the last three months of 2005 the international community gave a new impetus and new orientation to the treatment of avian flu in Vietnam. In 2005 the number of countries notifying H5N1 to the OIE increased dramatically and the virus reached Europe (with the first human cases in Europe occurring in Turkey in January 2006), increasing the pandemic threat for western countries. The same year the US Congress commissioned an assessment of the actions undertaken by the international community and by the main countries affected by the virus, including Vietnam. The report underlined numerous inadequacies in the surveillance and control of the virus. In line with the lessons learned from terrorist attacks, the US government was now convinced that it should not rely for homeland security solely on the surveillance and the protection of its own territory but that it had to increase its involvement at the international level to manage the sources of threat (Congressional Research Service [CRS] 2006). In September 2005 US President George W. Bush, addressing the United Nations World Summit, announced his country's decision to invest in and coordinate the formation of a new international partnership aimed at preventing an influenza pandemic. The President required all countries to be transparent on their epidemiological status (Bush 2005).

In addition, the appointment of a Senior United Nations System Coordinator for Avian and Human Influenza, Dr Nabarro, marked the globalisation of avian flu management. The WHO had already reinforced its presence in Vietnam at the time of SARS and it was now the turn of the FAO to widen the scope of its local activity. Bilateral cooperation developed primarily with the USA, as well as with Japan and New Zealand. NGOs also increased their presence in Vietnam (Academy for Educational Development, Association Vétérinaires sans Frontiè res and CARE). The UN agencies in Vietnam supervised the coordination of the donors and demanded in the middle of 2005 a greater involvement from the Vietnamese authorities: in particular, they asked for a direct and permanent line of communication with the Vietnamese prime minister (interview).

Vietnam came under increased pressure to attend to the pandemic threat. UN agencies asked for greater involvement from the Ministry of Health and the Vietnamese government was pressed to formulate a plan for human pandemic influenza preparedness and responses (the Red Book). This was the condition for obtaining a portion of the funds that the international community had committed to this cause (interview). The US government succeeded in imposing the presence, at the WHO office in Hanoi, of one of their military experts (from the Center for Disease Control and Prevention, Atlanta) against the will of the Vietnamese authorities (interview).

Vietnamese official government declarations became more frequent and the number of articles addressing the problem of avian flu in the press reached a new peak. The Prime Minister responded to UN pressure by addressing the nation for the first time since the beginning of the epizootic disease through an official telegram (Telegram no. 1686/TTg-NN), in which he announced reinforced measures to prevent and fight against avian flu. New laws were produced with the assistance of the FAO and OIE (MARD and MOH 2010). Moreover, Vietnam agreed to an experiment with a large-scale programme of poultry vaccination under the supervision of the FAO. As noted by international experts:

> At the beginning, Vietnam was a test; the rest of the world observed what happened. (International health expert, interview, 23 April 2008)

> Vietnam is a test and a model for controlling the disease. (Animal health expert, interview, 11 December 2007)

The participation of the private sector became more widely solicited. Through new regulations, new hygiene standards, a credit policy and even local tax policies, the government consistently promoted the development of a modern industrial poultry farming sector to the detriment of small-scale farming (ACI 2007). The state even passed the role of public health protection, traditionally its own responsibility (in particular in communist countries) onto the private sector, by a Health Ministry radio announcement in which people were told, 'If you don't want to catch the virus, buy your poultry at the supermarket'.

Why did Vietnam, a country with a reputation of strong adherence to national sovereignty, adopt the international framing of avian flu as a pandemic threat? And what was the extent of their compliance as a result of this adoption? Policy transfer studies (Delpeuch 2009) have shown that policy transfer is not a purely rational process oriented towards problem-solving. Many factors come into play when selecting and reframing imported policies, such as path dependency and cognitive and cultural factors.

Global risk instrumentalisation: from local to international issues

For the Vietnamese government, there were two political issues associated with avian flu management. As noted by a European expert:

Europe came here to analyse the problem in a scientific manner and to define a strategy based on science. But the objective of the Government is completely different! It aims at keeping stability in the country and to protect its reputation. (Interview, 27 April 2008)

The first phase of avian flu management proved to be beneficial for political stability, the centralisation of power and the promotion of a nationalist project. Following the deregulatory market reforms of 1986, provincial authorities gained new economic power and autonomy from the central government. Tuong (2010) has shown that the management of avian flu became an opportunity for the central government to affirm its authority, regardless of the local reality (as with the authoritarian imposition of massive culling measures). Central authorities used avian flu to blame local authorities for all mismanagement, pointing to their incompetence and corruption. The media presented the victory over the virus as a question of national honour and as popular mobilisation behind the Party against a new common enemy (Guénel and Klingberg 2010, Tuong 2010).

In contrast, during the second phase, the virus became an opportunity for Vietnam to consolidate a 20-year period of reintegration into the international diplomatic community. When H5N1 emerged, the USA, Vietnam's former enemy, was the last obstacle to its entry to the World Trade Organisation (WTO). Vietnam had yet to complete bilateral negotiations with the USA in order to obtain the status of a permanent normal trade relations (PNTR) nation from the US Congress (for more details see the US Association of Southeast Asian Nations Business Council 2006). These negotiations were part of a Vietnam–USA normalisation process depending on a number of key issues such as human rights, religious freedom, intellectual property rights and bird flu, as quoted by a US Congress Report (CRS 2005). There were successive visits by US officials to Vietnam in 2005 right up to the official visit by George Bush in November 2006. The US President closely linked Vietnam's entry to the WTO in 2006 to its successful handling of the pandemic threat (Embassy of the Republic of Vietnam 2006). In complying with the requirements of the USA and the international community, Vietnam seized the opportunity to present itself as a good global citizen:

This is a question which concerns not only this country, but all the world's countries. We must share this responsibility. Of course, the culling of chickens is a significant economic loss for the population, especially the poor, rural farmers . . . but the government is determined, and is also responsible to the rest of the world. (Ministry of Health representative, interview, 17 December 2007).

For one of the international experts involved since the beginning, the first phase in Vietnam's risk management was just a mistake:

For a long period, Vietnam has been seen as an enemy for the rest of the world. But during the last 15 years, the Government's objective has been to integrate the international community. When Vietnamese authorities understood the global dimension of the risk [HPAI], they reacted very quickly. Sure, they made some mistakes in 2004, but this did not last. (Interview, 24 April 2008)

Vietnam has been considered as being at the top of the class for complying with the requirements of the US administration and UN agencies, as confirmed by many of interviewees. But what were the real consequences of such compliance? Is it transformative cooperation or just lip-service?

A transformative cooperation for Vietnam?

Vietnam's compliance with international requirements brought risks to national sovereignty. The authorities adopted the framing of avian flu as a pandemic threat (that is as a risk of second modernity) and cooperated with the international community to manage a global manufactured uncertainty. They delivered transparent information on the outbreaks (according to our interviewees) and implemented a vaccination programme. Nevertheless, changes in Vietnamese policies have remained limited. Firstly, in the field many regulations adopted by the authorities were not applied or were applied for a short period only. For example, a ban on duck breeding has never been applied and live poultry markets, however much they were prohibited, have quickly resumed. According to MARD (2007), the implementation of one major decision (Decision 394 on biosecurity measures in the avian chain) has been limited. This discrepancy between norms and practices is a common feature of Vietnamese policy, according to Bao An and de Tréglodé (2004): it is a way for Vietnamese authorities to manage the contradictions of the country's development process: in this case, contradictions between the objective of international integration and the defence of national sovereignty.

Secondly, the authorities have recognised in their national strategy for avian flu (the Red Book) the need to rely on a wide web of stakeholders in order to manage the virus (international organisations, NGOs and the private sector). However, these stakeholders have been kept away from the decision-making process: they do not take part in the National Steering Committee (NSC) for Avian Influenza Disease Control and Prevention (established by Decision No. 13/2004/QD-TTg, dated 28 January 2004). This committee brings together representatives of ministries (including agriculture, health, trade, finance, transport and the environment) but does not include any representatives of civil society and its discussions are confidential. International and foreign organisations were also excluded from this committee. Debates with these organisations, and the coordination of their numerous activities, have been the role of the Partnership for Avian and Human Influenza (PAHI), created in 2005. According to one member of this partnership, this structure (the NSC and PAHI) clearly indicates the strategy of the Vietnamese authorities vis-á-vis cooperation and protection of national sovereignty:

> The functioning of the NSC demonstrates the sovereignty of Vietnam . . . The Vietnamese government affirms that it is completely open [and] ready to furnish any information, but that does not mean that international organisations can intervene in the NSC. The information is divulged via the PAHI to the international organisations. (Expert from PAHI, interview, 24 April 2008)

The democratic turn that, according to Beck, could be produced by global risks did not occur in Vietnam. And the capacity of transformations potentially induced by new global risks is shown to be limited compared to path dependency effects linked to Vietnam political characteristics.

Conclusion

As mentioned by one of our interviewees, a member of the PAHI:

> Vietnam plays the game because there is benefit to it. That is true that there are conditionalities linked to foreign aid. But donors are sometimes so naive. (Interview, 24 April 2008)

There were dual benefits for Vietnam at national and international levels. Modern risks are characterised by their potential for political destabilisation because they question the capacity of states to protect their citizens. But being global, they also question states' sovereignty as well as their reputation in the eyes of the other countries over their contribution to global goods.

However, in a very clever way, Vietnam exploited a number of opportunities associated with avian flu, both keeping the international community at a safe distance while adeptly navigating the unfamiliar path of global governance, changing its image in the world from that of a carrier of a global health risk to one of a good global citizen and finally consolidating the Communist heritage at a local level while advocating greater public health control via the market. This demonstrates the varieties of modernity. The Vietnamese representatives interviewed during this research were proud to underline that, in managing avian flu, Vietnam was not like China (because Vietnam remained accountable) nor was it like Laos (because Vietnam did not relinquish its sovereignty when the avian flu broke out), and that it was not like Indonesia (because Vietnam had always shown cooperation). But Vietnam's major success in avian flu management should be assessed from its primary result: Vietnam became the WTO's 150th member on 11 January 2007.

This Vietnamese case has been studied using the analytical framework offered by Beck's World at Risk theory. I have paid attention particularly to the constructed dimension of global risks, to the relations of definition as relations of domination and to the possibilities of instrumentalisation. This focus downplays global risks as structural factors that drive cosmopolitisation and democratisation. It also shows the community of fear to be a less powerful driver of cosmopolitisation than the community of trade.

Acknowledgements

This research was conducted with the support of the Gripavi and Ardigrip projects, funded by the French Ministry of Foreign and European Affairs and the French Ministry of Research.

References

Agrifood Consulting International (ACI) (2007) *The Economic Impact of Highly Pathogenic Avian Influenza*. Report prepared for FAO and WHO. Bethesda: ACI.

Bao An, Y. and de Tréglodé, B. (2004) Doi Moi et mutations du politique. In S. Dovert et de B. Tréglodé (eds) *Vietnam contemporain*. Paris: Institut de Recherche Sur l'Asie du Sud-Est Contemporaine.

Beck, U. (1992) *Risk Society: Towards a New Modernity*. London: Sage.

Beck, U. (2003) La société du risque globalisé revue sous l'angle de la menace terroriste, *Cahiers internationaux de sociologie*, 1, 114, 27–33.

Beck, U. (2009) *World at Risk*. Cambridge: Polity Press.

Beck, U. and Grande, E. (2010) Varieties of second modernity: the cosmopolitan turn in social and political theory and research, *British Journal of Sociology*, 61, 3, 409–43.

Boudia, S. and Jas, N. (2007) Risk and 'risk society' in historical perspective, *History and Technology*, 23, 4, 317–31.

Burgess, A. (2006) Editorial. The making of the risk-centred society and the limits of social risk research, *Health, Risk & Society*, 8, 4, 329–42.

Bush, G.W. (2005) Statement of H.E. Mr George W. Bush, President of the United States of America. 2005 UN World Summit, High Level Plenary Meeting of the 60th session of the General Assembly.

Available at http://www.un.org/webcast/summit2005/statements/usa050914.pdf (accessed 1 October 2012).

Calain, Ph. (2007) Exploring the international arena of global public health surveillance, *Health, Policy and Planning*, 22, 1, 2–12.

Calhoun, C. (2010) Beck, Asia and second modernity, *British Journal of Sociology*, 61, 3, 597–619.

Chang, K.-S. (2010) The second modern condition? Compressed modernity as internalized reflexive cosmopolitization, *British Journal of Sociology*, 61, 3, 446–64.

Congressional Research Service (CRS) (2005) The Vietnam–US normalization process. Congressional Research Service, Report for Congress. Available at http://www.fas.org/sgp/crs/row/IB98033.pdf (accessed 1 October 2012).

CRS (2006) U.S. and International responses to global spread of avian flu. Congressional Research Service, Report for Congress, RL33219. Available at http://www.fas.org/sgp/crs/misc/RL33219.pdf (accessed 1 October 2012).

Delpeuch, T. (2009) Comprendre la circulation internationale des solutions d'actions publiques: panorama des policy transfer studies, *Critique internationale*, 2, 43, 153–65.

Desvaux, S. and Figuié, M. (2011) Formal and informal surveillance systems. How to build bridges? *Bulletin de l'AEEMA*, 59–60, 352–55.

Dingwall, R. (1999) 'Risk society': the cult of theory and the millenium? *Social Policy and Administration*, 33, 4, 474–91.

Do Hien, (2004) Les relations internationales du Viêt Nam depuis 1991. In S. Dovert, B. de Tréglodé (eds) *Vietnam contemporain*. Paris: Institut de Recherche Sur l'Asie du Sud-Est Contemporaine.

Embassy of the Republic of Vietnam (2006) President Bush visits Vietnam. Available at http://vietnamembassy-usa.org/relations/president-bush-visits-vietnam (accessed 1 October 2012).

Figuié, M. and Fournier, T. (2008) Avian influenza in Vietnam: chicken-hearted consumers? *Risk Analysis*, 28, 2, 441–51.

Food and Agricultural Organization (FAO), World Organization for Animal Health (OIE), World Health Organization (WHO) (2004) Unprecedented spread of avian influenza requires broad collaboration. FAO/OIE/WHO call for international assistance. Press Release. WHO media center. Available at http://www.who.int/mediacentre/news/releases/2004/pr7/en/ (accessed 1 October 2012).

FAO, OIE, WHO, United Nations System Influenza Coordination, United Nations Children's Fund and the World Bank (2008) Contributing to One World, One Health. Available at ftp://ftp.fao.org/docrep/fao/011/aj137e/aj137e00.pdf (accessed 1 October 2012).

Gilbert, C. (ed.) (2007) *Les Crises sanitaires de grande Ampleur: Un nouveau défi?* Paris: Institut national des Hautes Etudes de Sécurité (INHES).

Guénel, A. and Klingberg, S. (2010) Press Coverage of Bird flu epidemic in Vietnam. In Liew Kai Khiun (ed.) *Liberalizing, Feminizing and Popularizing Health Communications in Asia*. Farnham: Ashgate.

Han, S.-J. and Shim, Y.-H. (2010) Redefining second modernity for East Asia: a critical assessment, *British Journal of Sociology*, 61, 3, 465–87.

Kyung-Sup, C. (2010) The second modern condition? Compressed modernity as internalized reflexive cosmopolitization, *British Journal of Sociology*, 61, 3, 444–64.

Ministry of Agriculture and Rural Development (MARD) (2007) *Provincial summary reports on implementing Prime Minister Decision 394/QD-TTG*. Hanoi: Ministry of Agriculture and Rural Development.

MARD and Ministry of Health (MOH) (2010) *Avian and pandemic influenza. Vietnam's experience*. Hanoi: Ministry of Agriculture and Rural Development and Ministry of Health.

Méric, J., Pesqueux, Y. and Solé, A. (2009) *La 'société du risque'. Analyse et critique*. Paris: Economica.

Mythen, G. (2007) Reappraising the risk society thesis, *Current Sociology*, 55, 6, 793–813.

Poultry Diseases Network (2007) David Nabarro warns of an inevitable influenza pandemic. 18 September. Available at http://www.poultrydiseases.net/online/index.php?option=com_content&task=view&id=172&Itemid=54 (accessed 1 October 2012).

Renn, O. (2008) *Risk Governance: Coping with Uncertainty in a Complex World*. London: Earthscan.

Scoones, I. (eds) (2010) *Avian Influenza. Science, Policy and Politics*. London: Earthscan.

Taylor-Gooby, P and Zinn, J.O. (eds) (2006) *Risk in Social Science*. Oxford: Oxford University Press.

Tuong, V. (2010) Power, politics and accountability: Vietnam's response to avian influenza. In Scoones (ed.) *Avian Influenza. Science, Policy and Politics*. London: Earthscan.

US Association of Southeast Asian Nations Business Council (2006) Vietnam WTO accession: permanent normal trade relations. Available at http://www.usvtc.org/trade/wto/PNTRmemo.pdf (accessed 1 October 2012).

Vallat, B. (2007) Protecting the world from emerging diseases linked to globalization. Editorial. OIE Bulletins Online, 2/2007. Available at http://www.oie.int/for-the-media/editorials/detail/article/protecting-the-world-from-emerging-diseases-linked-to-globalisation/ (accessed 1 October 2012).

Vietnam Development Report (2004) *Poverty 2004. Vietnam Consultative Group (ADB, AusAID, DFID, GTZ, JICA, Save the Children UK, UNDP, World Bank)*. Hanoi: ADB.

World Health Organization (WHO) (2005a) Introduction to the IHR 2005, World Health Organization, *IHR brief*, 1. Available at http://www.who.int/ihr/ihrbrief1en.pdf (accessed 1 October 2012).

WHO (2005a) Outbreak communication. World Health Organization handbook for journalists: Influenza Pandemic. Available at http://www.who.int/csr/don/Handbook_influenza_pandemic_dec05.pdf (accessed 1 October 2012).

WHO (2005b) International Health regulations. Notification and other reporting requirements under the IHR (2005), IHR brief no. 2. Available at http://www.who.int/ihr/about/en/index.html (accessed 1 October 2012).

WHO (2007a) The world health report 2007. A safer future: global public health security in the 21st century. Available at http://www.who.int/whr/2007/en/index.html (accessed 1 October 2012).

WHO (2007b) World health report 2007 press kit. Presentation. Available at http://www.who.int/whr/2007/media_centre/slides_en.pdf (accessed 6 October 2012).

WHO (2012) Influenza: cumulative number of confirmed human cases of avian influenza A(H5N1) reported to WHO. Table 26 March. Available at http://www.who.int/influenza/human_animal_interface/H5N1_cumulative_table_archives/en/index.html (accessed 6 October 2012).

World Organization for Animal Health (OIE) (2009) One World, One Health. *OIE Bulletins online*, 2/2009. Available at http://www.oie.int/fileadmin/Home/eng/Publications_%26_Documentation/docs/pdf/Bull_2009-2-ENG.pdf (accessed 1 October 2012).

World Organization for Animal Health (OIE) (2012) *WAHID Interface. Country information*. Available at http://www.oie.int/wahis_2/public/wahid.php/Countryinformation/Animalsituation (accessed 29 October 2012).

7

The politics of securing borders and the identities of disease
Rosemary C.R. Taylor

How do nations respond to health threats perceived to originate beyond their borders? This question is explored by examining efforts in three member states of the European Union (EU) – France, Britain and Germany, to contain the spread into their territories of two diseases, human immunodeficiency virus/acquired immune deficiency syndrome (HIV/AIDS) and tuberculosis (TB). The policy cases are representative of broader measures taken to meet emergent public health threats posed by peoples and products. Both HIV/AIDS and TB are communicable diseases, posing a threat to public health and generating cross-border problems associated with migration. I argue that the making of policies to contain them cannot be understood without an examination of the identities they acquire over time, and that these disease identities shape decision-makers' views about the threat posed by these diseases, what should be done to contain them and specifically, what measures should be adopted towards screening at the border.

The cases

HIV/AIDS and TB are problems of increasing concern in Europe. National surveillance systems and local studies have detected a high rate of HIV among migrants and ethnic and racial minorities (Del Amo *et al.* 2004). European monitors note that 'many HIV infections have been diagnosed in immigrants from countries with generalised HIV epidemics' (Hamers *et al.* 2006) and the incidence of HIV/AIDS in the EU is increasingly affected by international travel and migration.

One-third of the world's population is thought to be infected with latent TB. Its resurgence in many industrialised nations is related to three factors: the emergence of drug-resistant strains, its appearance among people with damaged immune systems and its incidence among the 'foreign-born': people from countries with a high level of the disease (Klaudt 2000). Unlike HIV, TB is not a new disease: measures to cope with infected persons have long been incorporated into national and international health regulations. Nevertheless, its re-emergence prompted the World Health Organization (WHO) to declare a 'world emergency' in 1993 and Europe has seen significant increases in some metropolitan centres,

Pandemics and Emerging Infectious Diseases: The Sociological Agenda, First Edition. Edited by Robert Dingwall, Lily M. Hoffman and Karen Staniland. Chapters © 2013 The Authors. Book Compilation © 2013 Foundation for the Sociology of Health & Illness / John Wiley & Sons Ltd.

such as London, where TB rates have doubled over the last two decades (Rose *et al.* 2001). Resource-poor Eastern European countries have fared much worse (Walls and Shingadia 2007).

The problematic

The measures taken to contain HIV/AIDS and TB centre on the notification, quarantine, surveillance, screening or treatment of people. All these measures challenge democratic societies. They question long-accepted boundaries between the public and private spheres by asking public officials to concern themselves with the most personal of actions. They put pressure on conventionally accepted liberties, including freedom of movement and from arbitrary incarceration. How do national governments arrive at measures designed to protect public health that challenge such liberties? How does each government deal with the fact that efforts to contain health threats seen to be coming from abroad may entail discrimination against particular categories of people?

The European Union

I consider three national cases: Germany, Britain and France. All are known for taking different approaches to public health. Germany has long been the 'greenest' nation, where the regulation of products and health has been strict. Britain and France are often seen as laggards, despite the market orientation of the former and extensive state intervention in the latter, but they, too, are shifting their policies in response to new threats. Both experienced scandals in the 1990s over their perceived failures to contain threats to public health – bovine spongiform encephalopathy and variant Creutzfeldt–Jakob disease in Britain and the transmission of HIV via blood and blood products in France. All three nations have recently tightened restrictions in the face of increased immigration. They provide good cases in which to examine how nations with different approaches to securing public health have coped with these new challenges.

All are also core member states of the EU, where we see a dynamic in which national experts contend over the most appropriate way to define problems and solutions. Limiting the movement of people or products across borders is an established method for containing diseases but such 'fortress' strategies (Collin and Lee 2003) pose particular dilemmas in Europe because they run counter to the EU's pursuit of four freedoms – the free movement of people, goods, services and capital. When applied, they have often increased political tensions and inspired trade battles among the member states (Judt 2001).

Protecting borders

The measures nations favour to keep communicable diseases out of their territories are to test, screen and examine. The rationale is usually

- surveillance, to see how far an epidemic has spread
- to make people aware that they have a disease, on the assumption that this knowledge will lead to behavioural change
- to allow for triage and treatment

Testing is also undertaken for exclusionary reasons; however, as Figures 1 and 2 indicate, not all nations conduct testing, do so in the same fashion or use the results to exclude people. Given the EU's permissive stance – 'member states *may* require medical screening on public health grounds' (European Union 2003: 21, my emphasis), which does not prevent member states from taking whatever measures they deem appropriate – it is curious that three core nations have done virtually the same thing with regard to TB and HIV. All screen and test for TB but, with a few local exceptions, do not screen or test migrants for HIV.

Explaining variations in screening across diseases

Why have these nations taken a stance toward screening for HIV so different from that employed for TB? Two broad approaches emerge from the literature as likely explanations. The first is *an approach from health science*, which assumes that policy responses are driven largely by data on the incidence and severity of the threat, calibrated to existing scientific means for testing and treatment. While such factors matter at a general level, they do not offer much explanatory power in this case. Regulations concerning TB were initially established at the end of the 19th century, when all three countries had a high incidence of the disease, but the number of cases declined substantially during the 20th century with few corresponding regulatory changes. Much later, when HIV was identified as the cause of AIDS, the disease was quickly seen as a transnational epidemic. A health science logic would predict that countries already screening for TB would also screen for HIV, but Britain, France and Germany did not.

Similarly, a health science perspective would predict that, when the danger of TB receded in industrialised countries and then re-emerged, changes in screening practices would mirror the waning and waxing of the threat, but they did not. Of course, policy might be conditioned by the science associated with screening. Again, experience contradicts the expectation: once a test for AIDS was devised, it was relatively easy to administer, while testing

	Visitors and tourists	Immigrants	Refugees	Asylum seekers
France	No	Yes – Chest X-ray for medical certificate for long-stay visas and residence permits; after 'loi Sarkozy', 25 November 2003, only for non-EU citizens	Yes – at reception/holding centres (Norredam *et al.* 2006). Following determination of latent TB: no action except under15 year-olds sent to hospital for preventive treatment (Coker *et al.* 2004)	
Germany	No	Yes – including Aussiedler (Feil *et al.* 2004)	Yes	
UK	No (unless visit is longer than 6 months)	Yes – depending on country of origin: 67 countries with high incidence of TB require screening before entry into the UK (UK Home Office 2012)	Yes – at reception/induction centres (Norredam *et al.* 2006)	
EU	No		Member states may require applicants to be medically screened on public health grounds (EU 2003)	

Figure 1 *National practices for screening/excluding visitors and migrants for tuberculosis (TB)*

	Visitors and Tourists	Immigrants	Refugees	Asylum Seekers
France	No mandatory testing (Klein 2001) No HIV-related restrictions on entry, stay or residence (Wiessner and Lemmen 2002)	Medical exam required for stay > 3 months; may include HIV test Residence cannot be refused solely based on positive serology for HIV[1]	No mandatory testing If a person needs medical treatment not available in their country of origin, this may be grounds for a residence permit (Wiessner and Lemmen 2002)	
Germany	Medical exams not required to enter the country (Klein 2001) No routine testing or regulations for PLHIV	No restrictions on immigrants Officials may refuse a residence permit if applicant has a contagious disease; HIV considered a contagious disease under federal law[2] *Except Bavaria:* HIV test can be required for Non-EU citizens staying for >180 days (Lazarus et al. 2010)	No restrictions on refugees	HIV tests routinely performed on asylum seekers Positive results do not affect application decision but may make applicant eligible for immediate medical care[3] *Saxony and New Brandenburg:* HIV test required for asylum seekers (Lazarus et al. 2010)
U.K.	No mandatory testing No HIV-related restrictions on entry, stay or residence (Wiessner and Lemmen 2002) PLHIV cannot be automatically excluded; however, the Department of Public Health may exclude individuals they consider risks to public health (Klein 2001) Known PLHIV must prove they are able to pay for treatment during their visit (Klein 2001)	Ability to support self and family taken into account when granting residence[4] Non-EU citizens seeking to reside for more than 6 months must report for medical inspection; HIV seropositivity will not exclude applicants	No HIV-related restrictions	Asylum may be granted on medical grounds, including HIV/AIDS, under the principle of *non-refoulement* but only under exceptional circumstances and in cases of extreme illness (Ingram 2008) Neither requesting nor disclosing positive status will adversely affect asylum claims (NAM 2010)
E.U.	The EU explicitly condemns HIV-related entry restrictions[5] EU citizens can travel freely within the EU except in: UK, Ireland, Denmark (HIV positivity has no impact)	Member states may, within 3 months of a person's arrival, require persons entitled to the right of residence to take a free medical exam to certify that they do not have any of the *diseases of epidemic[6] potential*	All member states abide by the principle of *non-refoulement*	The European Court of Human Rights has ruled that in some cases asylum must be granted to HIV-positive individuals on humanitarian grounds; however, the circumstances must be exceptional Member states may require medical screening on public health grounds (EU 2003)

Figure 2 *National practices for screening/excluding human immunodeficiency virus HIV-positive visitors and migrants.*

[1] *Government of France 1987.*

[2] *If people living with human immunodeficiency virus (PLHIV) show symptoms of HIV, are required to take a medical exam and are found to be HIV-positive, residence can be refused (Klein 2001).*

[3] *If HIV medication or care is unavailable in applicant's country of origin, applicant may be able to argue for asylum based on non-refoulement, the protection given to refugees from being returned to places where their lives or freedoms could be threatened (Marcus, 2000).*

[4] *HIV/AIDS is not considered a disease that warrants public health exclusion but PLHIV may be considered unable to support themselves and their families, which could lead to exclusion (Klein 2001).*

[5] *European Commission (2009).*

[6] *Diseases of epidemic potential include: anthrax, dengue, HIV/AIDS, malaria, measles, tuberculosis (TB), multi-drug resistant TB (World Health Organization 2008).*

for TB remains protracted and difficult. Although logical, the approach from health science does not offer much purchase over this comparative case.

A policy legacies approach has been advanced by Baldwin (2005) and Weir and Skocpol (1985). In an effort to explain AIDS strategies in several countries, Baldwin argues that national differences are path dependent, driven by templates for coping with disease set in the context of 19th century epidemics such as cholera and syphilis. This approach is more sensitive to political determinants but implies that countries that test for TB should test for AIDS. Thus, it cannot explain why Britain, France and Germany do not.

Disease identities

To explain the different approaches of these countries to screening migrants and other travellers for TB and HIV, I suggest that we need to see diseases in more sociological terms, as phenomena whose sufferers acquire certain 'identities'. These identities are typically forged at the time when the disease acquires prominence in public discourse and, like the stereotypes associated with minority groups, they are slow to change and difficult to dispel. Thus, identities associated with a disease shaped in a specific historical context travel forward through time where they remain influential even in new contexts.

The idea of a 'disease identity' draws on several lines of inquiry. Medical sociologists (Brown 1995, Conrad and Barker 2010, Ingleby 1982) have argued that disease is 'socially constructed'. The implications are several: this perspective questions the assumption that 'disease classification is based solely on objective and discrete clinical and epidemiological criteria' (Aronowitz 1999: 12), and highlights the negotiations among multiple social actors, including, but not limited to, doctors and patients, over the meaning of diagnoses and disease labels. In this view, diseases do not simply exist in nature; over time, they are discussed, debated and established as 'agreed-upon disease categories' (Rosenberg 2002: 237).

Most historians and social scientists would not quarrel with this claim. A substantial body of literature now describes the emergence of disease entities in different times and places. However, as Dwyer wrote memorably of epilepsy, how exactly such categories are generated is a story sometimes 'easier to tell than to explain' (1992: 251). Some accounts privilege technological development and competition among medical specialties (Wailoo 1999); others reference broader cultural and institutional changes. The important point is that, whatever the process, diseases acquire a distinctive identity as well as a diagnostic label as they emerge; in Rosenberg's terms the disease is 'invested with a unique configuration of social characteristics, and thus triggers disease-specific responses' (1992: xviii).

The formation of disease identities is a complex discursive process, constructed by a variety of political, professional and cultural actors, in which advances in science or medicine are by no means the arbiter of how a disease is understood. Some disease identities are contested. Once afflicted, the sick fight to define who they are, shunning the label of 'victim', for example, and attempt to refashion identities for themselves using available repertoires of symbolic and material resources. But the latter are composed of categories collectively created over time by negotiations among different groups, ranging from medical professionals and government officials to artists and journalists. Disease identities are thus collective constructs. They may emerge in reaction to national histories, but they are also forged from local practices and debated in international forums.

The importance of such identities, I argue, lies in the ways in which they inform the policies adopted to address the disease. As Rosenberg (1992: xviii) has suggested, 'once articulated and accepted, disease identities become "actors" in a complex network of social negotiations'. Images of who has a disease are inextricable from the disease itself in the eyes of the public and of policymakers, and colour the approaches the latter take towards controlling that disease. These considerations are likely to have particular relevance for decisions, not only about the best way to cope with an epidemic, but about how to balance ancillary issues, such as how much to infringe on personal liberties and whom to contain or quarantine.

In what follows I argue that the identity of a disease conditions how policymakers approach epidemics, discussing, first, how TB and AIDS acquired their contemporary identities and, then, how these identities affected the policy process.

Tuberculosis: diseased immigrants and recalcitrant patients

When TB was first identified in the 19th century, it was described as the 'captain of death'. Because little was known about its causes and cure, it was portrayed in terms shaped more by national mythologies than scientific facts. Sontag (1978) has argued that, when the causes of a disease are unknown, it will be described in terms reflecting those things of which society is most afraid. In the case of TB, those fears centred on the 'economic man' required by capitalism, a form of economic organisation that requires investment, discipline and saving, and fears reckless or spendthrift behaviour. Whether or not one is convinced by Sontag's argument, her characterisation of the imagery attaching to this disease in 19th century Europe is accurate: TB was portrayed as a disease of unbridled passion, associated with overly sensitive people of artistic temperament.

Treatments based on finding a dry climate or taking a sea voyage, intended for a European elite, were soon institutionalised in the form of the sanatorium. However, the sanatorium was only briefly the refuge of the wealthy. As more segments of the population were afflicted it became a place to isolate the sick and provide them with moral education (Feldberg 1995). Scholars debate the degree to which sanatoria served to discipline and control the working class (Bashford 2004). Condrau's recent appraisal concludes that 'the available sanitorium case studies confirm that they were no concentration camps; equally they were no cosy Magic Mountains either' (2010: 92).

At the end of World War II the use of the Bacillus Calmette–Guérin vaccine by relief organisations in Eastern Europe was credited with preventing a major TB epidemic and adopted in many European nations. In 1951 isoniazid, discovered in 1912, was found to be effective against TB. With the incidence of TB declining, and confident that drug therapy would soon vanquish it entirely, many societies began to dismantle the institutions of TB management (Smith-Nonini 2004).

Their satisfaction was temporary. By the late 1980s the incidence of TB began to rise in many countries and the growth of multi-drug-resistant TB (MDRTB) cast the disease as a 're-emerging' threat (Nolan 1997). Moreover, the new TB had acquired further negative connotations. Reflecting a widespread consensus, Barnes could write that:

> the recent resurgence of tuberculosis in the United States and other industrialized countries has taken place among certain clearly identifiable communities and 'risk groups': homeless people, drug addicts, prison inmates, poor immigrants, migrant farm workers, the elderly, and people with HIV infection and AIDS (1995: 3).

In the 21st century public mind, TB is associated with poverty, homelessness and, above all, migrants. Non-citizens are disproportionately represented among its sufferers in Europe, but there is considerable debate about whether migrants develop these diseases in their countries of origin or after their arrival. Whether immigrants are transmitting infection to the native-born population has become a politically sensitive issue. In the case of people with MDRTB, the relevant imagery often references carelessness and self-destructive behaviour: the disease becomes drug-resistant because patients stopped treatment too soon – they are 'non-compliant' (see Lerner 1997). Not only have they condemned themselves to an arduous regime of treatment but, even worse, they have become a danger to society. In more than one country suggestions have been made that they should be forcibly detained or at a minimum treated under close supervision.

TB has now been stripped of mystery: its aetiology is well understood and treatments exist, although they are lengthy and not always successful. To be sure, it is not the same disease as it was in the second half of the 19th century. As Cunningham (2002) argues, at different times, all diseases are construed and created by different ways of thinking. Nevertheless, people suffering from TB have been consistently characterised as life's unfortunates, at best, and portrayed in increasingly negative terms as weak in both character and constitution, even when gifted, as poor, immigrant victims with few resources and, finally, as negligent and dangerous carriers.

People with AIDS (PWA)

AIDS emerged in a different time – without a prehistory. Although its origins are disputed, it was first publicly identified as a new phenomenon in the United States in 1981. Initial reactions were similar across the globe: fear, consternation at the unknowns and discrimination against people who developed the opportunistic infections to which their damaged immune systems were prey.

This initial perception changed quickly in the developed world because gay men, who figured most prominently in the US epidemiology, had recently thrown off the stigma attached to homosexuality and become a vocal minority demanding the same civil rights as others on the basis of identity (see Bayer 1989, Shilts 2007). After 10 years of gay liberation it was difficult for members of this community to abandon sexual practices that were now classified as dangerous. Fierce debates over privacy, rights and health followed. However, gay men eventually became a mobilised interest group with regard to HIV/AIDS, winning a series of battles over issues such as contact tracing, participation in clinical trials and faster dissemination of drugs. In symbolic terms, these efforts culminated in the US with the incorporation of AIDS into the Americans with Disabilities Act.

In many parts of Europe, similar gay rights groups developed during the 1980s. Even in France, where a sharper line between the public and the private muted the movement's impact, it had a discernible presence and such groups were vociferous in Britain and Germany. AIDS also emerged during a period when many societies were being influenced by a transnational human rights discourse promoted by a host of non-governmental organisations. Human rights became a rallying cry with wide public resonance (Buergenthal 2006). Accordingly, informed consent became the sine qua non of HIV testing; even when AIDS was transformed into a more 'manageable' disease and testing guidelines were fiercely debated, this principle was not discarded (Bayer and Edington 2009).

Thus, AIDS, too, acquired a certain identity by virtue of the context in which it came to public attention. The image of the PWA that emerged in the developed democracies was a person who had rights that should be upheld. Given the early perception of AIDS, when the behaviour assumed to have 'caused' it was censored and its practitioners stigmatised, this is surprising, and AIDS still carries a stigma in many developing nations. Nevertheless, despite fear-mongering campaigns, anti-gay prejudice and tabloid hysteria (Garfield 1994), PWAs won both benefits and protection. The practices of European nations with regard to the treatment of HIV/AIDS vary, but their refusal to require mandatory HIV testing of immigrants can be attributed in significant part to these dimensions of the disease identity.

By contrast, sufferers from TB have never acquired the same status in the popular imagination. The longstanding stereotypes associated with that disease lingered. No TB acronyms have emerged to parallel the terms that mobilised groups around HIV/AIDS, such as PWA and PLHIV (people living with HIV). Internationally, there has been some attention to the rights of people suffering from TB (see, for example, Coker 2000). A patients' charter for tuberculosis care was eventually drawn up in 2006 by the World Care Council based in France and India and adopted by WHO. But it has been promoted mostly by volunteers and community-based organisations and is not yet widely accepted by national TB programmes (Raviglione 2007). There are no national or international groups of people with TB pushing to have their rights respected, and no equivalent for them of the AIDS quilt to mourn and memorialise those who have died. Thus, for the purposes of entry into the nations considered here, you may be an immigrant first, and a sick immigrant second, but your fate will depend to a great extent on the disease you carry.

Disease identities and the making of policy

Once established, however, disease identities are not inscribed automatically on the policies of nations. As Welshman (2006) demonstrates in the case of TB in Britain in the 1950s and 1960s, devising a screening strategy was a complex process and many factors – moral panics, a perceived demand for labour, the view of professional bodies – were involved in it. This leads to my second question: how do disease identities come to inform what countries do about screening immigrants?

Here, institutional structures become important because they allow for the promotion of national, regional and supranational cultural repertoires that are often biased in favour of or against particular disease identities. In this context the Bavarian exception is instructive. Bavaria requires routine HIV testing for all foreigners wishing to stay for more than six months, with the exception of EU citizens and Swiss nationals (Lazarus *et al.* 2010). These policies contrast with the generally liberal position of the West German (Pollak 1990) and then the German governments.

Bavaria's position emerged from its efforts in the 1980s to address AIDS with a repressive set of measures, which included prosecuting individuals for practising unsafe sex (Borneman 1987), requiring prostitutes to use condoms and stipulating that HIV-positive individuals must inform their sexual partners and doctors. The Bavarian government argued that it was treating AIDS like any other communicable disease, under the terms of the Federal Epidemics Control Act 1961 (Frankenberg 1990) and pressured the federal government to adopt a comprehensive programme of compulsory testing of prostitutes, drug users, prisoners, civil servants and foreigners (Frankenberg 1988). However, the Ministry of Health, Conference of State Ministers of Health and major political parties resisted this campaign and in 1987 an isolated Bavaria crafted a set of AIDS policies to be implemented within its own boundaries.

How is this to be explained? Baldwin argues that electoral manoeuvering played some role: 'the Christian Socialists hoped to distinguish themselves from their coalition allies during the spring 1987 elections' (2005: 57). Individual politicians were influential: Peter Gauweiler, the Bavarian Secretary for Internal Affairs, pursued a determined crusade against the sexual and moral deviants whom he saw as generating a world epidemic of AIDS. However, I place more weight on the influence of a distinctive regional political culture that promoted a disease identity that diverged from the one associated with AIDS elsewhere in Europe.

Bavaria's political culture, fostered by the Christian Social Union (CSU) that has governed Bavaria almost continuously since 1946, is Catholic, conservative and patriotic (Hepburn 2008, Sutherland 2001). It has been friendly neither to immigrants, seeking 'to preserve and protect the Bavarian Heimat from foreign cultures, especially those outside the EU' (Hepburn 2009: 518), nor to homosexuals. In 2005 the CSU filed a lawsuit in Germany's Federal Constitutional Court to prevent homosexual couples from being allowed to adopt children (Böhringer and Verbeet, 2005).

Given this regional culture, it is not surprising that Bavaria's positions on AIDS reflected a different disease identity. But here we also see the mediating roles that institutional structures play in the translation of disease identities into policy. On the one hand, Germany's federal polity allowed for the development of regional political cultures that conditioned disease identities and, on the other hand, by allocating authority over health- related policy to both federal government and the states (*Länder*) (Freeman 1992), it allowed Bavaria to implement a separate set of AIDS policies. Bavaria did not have the authority to legislate them but implemented them using administrative orders (Pollak 1990). A regionally specific conception of HIV-positive individuals could be developed and expressed in policy.

Europe and the collective imaginary

Supranational institutions can also play this type of mediating role. I have argued that explaining why European states took different approaches towards would-be entrants suffering from HIV/AIDS and TB requires understanding how those two diseases became associated with particular identities when the epidemic first came to public attention. In general, the liberal treatment accorded immigrants with HIV/AIDS is linked to an identity they acquired under the influence of a transnational human rights discourse prominent at the time the disease became an epidemic. However, this human rights discourse was not all-powerful: some states outside Europe continued to test immigrants for HIV/AIDS, including the United States, which stopped only in 2010. Therefore, something more must have been at work in Europe.

In this case, the decisive factor was the presence of the EU – a supranational institutional regime – determined to promote, not only the free movement of people, but a concept of 'European citizenship'. The rise of the AIDS epidemic coincided almost exactly with EU initiatives to create a common European citizenship in the wake of the Single European Act of 1986 and the negotiation of the Schengen Accords on the free movement of people. The effect of these initiatives was to blur the line that might once have been drawn between national citizens and the nationals of other states. It drew Europeans into a protracted process dominated by 'rights talk' and framed issues of migration in rights-based terms at just that point when decisions about whether to require HIV testing were being made. EU initiatives to construct a European citizenship biased national policy-making against such a requirement.

Thus, the importance of the EU lies not simply in how it shuffles jurisdiction over policymaking, but in how it transforms, at the level of ideas, what I will call the European collective imaginary. The collective imaginary[1] of a society is composed of the narratives that tie its past to its future, and specify who belongs to the community and what its members owe one another, much like the 'moral economies' of E.P. Thompson. The EU has long seen its mission as one of promoting a new collective imaginary.

Collective imaginaries affect policy in multiple ways. It can be through the mechanisms Soysal describes where immigrant groups mobilise to bolster their claims by drawing upon universal principles of human rights (Soysal 2001, 2004). Ideas can also be 'translated' from a global or European imaginary by intermediaries who 'negotiate between local, regional, national, and global systems of meaning' (Merry 2006: 39). As Favell notes:

> It is possible to show that at a certain point in time – and for contingent political reasons – the ideals and values carried within the idiom of citizenship [have] a decisive influence on the shape and outcome of the politics (1997: 174).

However, these imaginaries are not an immutable feature of societies but an evolving reservoir of myths, narratives and distinctions. As policymakers and others draw on some images and narratives rather than others, they subtly transmute what they can accomplish in the future, even as they accomplish something in the present. Herein lies the concept's wider significance. Just as the European collective imaginary of the 1980s and early 1990s influenced governments' approaches to migrants with AIDS, so it can be expected to influence their approaches to other kinds of health threats, conditioning how decision-makers treat disease carriers, what kinds of collective mobilization will be possible in the event of a disease outbreak, and the potential for panic and social disorder.

Conclusion

I have used the cases of HIV/AIDS and TB to explore broader theories about why governments take different approaches to epidemics. Influential perspectives based on health science and policy legacies gave little purchase. For a deeper insight, I have suggested we explore the role of disease identities, arguing that all diseases acquire an identity in the form of particular images of those who suffer from them, and that these identities endure over time and inform the policies governments adopt, especially where corollary judgments must be made about the rights of the individual.

Of course, there are limits to such arguments. Governments try, often conscientiously, to be attentive to the science of an emerging epidemic and their actions are influenced by other factors, such as electoral pressures and the evolving views of epistemic communities. We might expect the identities associated with a disease to be more important with regard to health threats seen to be moving across borders, which invariably require some interpretation of what is 'foreign' and what is 'familiar'. But the broader point is that public health policies are rarely made without reference to the wider context of citizenship regimes and the collective imaginaries that embody them (Favell 1997, Jenson 2007). Thus, there is value in considering how diseases acquire an identity and how such identities condition the positions taken by policymakers on complex trade-offs between privacy and the public health, civil rights and the public welfare and how foreigners, as compared to citizens, are treated.

Acknowledgements

I wish to thank Natalie Sullivan and Jeffrey Bower (2003) for research assistance and Susan Bell, Jim Ennis, Peter Hall, Margitta Maetzke, two anonymous reviewers and the editors of this special issue for insightful comments. I also benefited from the response of colleagues to earlier drafts presented at the Bremen International Graduate School of Social Sciences, the Juan March Institute, Madrid, the Sociology Department, Tufts University and the Hanse-Wissenschaftskolleg, Delmenhorst where the author was a fellow in autumn 2010. The latter's support is gratefully acknowledged.

Note

1   See essays in Hall and Lamont (2009) for an elaboration of this concept.

References

Aronowitz, R.A. (1999) *Making Sense of Illness: Science, Society, and Disease.* Cambridge: Cambridge University Press.

Baldwin, P. (2005) *Disease and Democracy: The Industrialized World Faces AIDS.* Berkeley and Los Angeles: University of California Press.

Barnes, D.S. (1995) *The Making of a Social Disease: Tuberculosis in Nineteenth-Century France.* Berkeley and Los Angeles: University of California Press.

Bashford, A. (2004) Tuberculosis: governing healthy citizens. In Bashford, A. (ed.) *Imperial Hygiene: a Critical History of Colonialism, Nationalism and Public Health.* New York: Palgrave Macmillan.

Bayer, R. (1989) *Private Acts, Social Consequences: AIDS and the Politics of Public Health.* New York: Free Press.

Bayer, R. and Edington, C. (2009) HIV testing, human rights, and global AIDS policy: exceptionalism and its discontents, *Journal of Health Politics, Policy and Law*, 34, 3, 301–23.

Böhringer, C. and Verbeet, M. (2005) Bavarian family values: state seeks to stop federal gay adoption rights. 29 April. *Spiegel Online International*, 17. Available at http://www.spiegel.de/international/spiegel/bavarian-family-values-state-seeks-to-stop-federal-gay-adoption-rights-a-353942.html

Borneman, J. (1987) AIDS in the two Berlins. *October: Journal of Art, Politics, Culture*, 43, Winter, 223–37.

Brown, P. (1995) Naming and framing: the social construction of diagnosis and illness, *Journal of Health and Social Behavior*, 36, Special issue, 34–52.

Buergenthal, T. (2006) The evolving international human rights system, *The American Journal of International Law*, 100, 4, 783–807.

Coker, R., Bell, A., Pitman, R., Hayward, A., et al. (2004) Screening programmes for tuberculosis in new entrants across Europe, *The International Journal of Tuberculosis and Lung Disease*, 8, 8, 1022–6.

Coker, R.J. (2000) *From Chaos to Coercion: Detention and the Control of Tuberculosis.* Basingstoke: Palgrave Macmillan.

Collin, J. and Lee, K. (2003) *Globalisation and Transborder Health Risk in the UK, Case Studies in Tobacco Control and Population Mobility.* London: Nuffield Trust.

Condrau, F. (2010) Beyond the total institution: towards a reinterpretation of the tuberculosis sanitorium. In Worboys, M. and Condrau, F. (eds), *Tuberculosis Then and Now: Perspectives on the History of an Infectious Disease.* Montreal and Kingston: McGill-Queen's University Press.

Conrad, P. and Barker, K.K. (2010) The social construction of illness, *Journal of Health and Social Behavior*, 51, 1, S67–79.

Cunningham, A. (2002) Identifying disease in the past: cutting the Gordian knot, *Asclepio*, 54, 1, 13–34.

Del Amo, J., Broring, G., Hamers, F.F. and Infuso, A. et al. (2004) Monitoring HIV/AIDS in Europe's migrant communities and ethnic minorities, *AIDS*, 18, 14, 1867–73.

Dwyer, E. (1992) Stories of epilepsy, 1880–1930. In Rosenberg, C.E. and Golden, J. (eds), *Framing Disease: Studies in Cultural History.* New Brunswick: Rutgers University Press.

European Commission (2009) Communication from the Commission to the European Parliament, the Council, the European Economic and Social Committee and the Committee of the Regions –

Combating HIV/AIDS in the European Union and neighbouring countries, 2009–2013. COM/2009/0569 final. Brussels: Commission of the European Communities.

European Union (2003) Council Directive 2003/9/EC: laying down minimum standards for the reception of asylum seekers, *Official Journal of the European Union*, 6.2.2003, L 31/18–25.

Favell, A. (1997) Citizenship and immigration: pathologies of a progressive philosophy, *Journal of Ethnic and Migration Studies*, 23, 2, 173–95.

Feil, F., Dreesman, J. and Steffens, I. (2004) Tuberculosis screening of *Aussiedler* at the Friedland border immigration centre, Germany, *Euro Surveillance*, 9, 2, 50–1.

Feldberg, G.D. (1995) *Disease and Class: Tuberculosis and the Shaping of Modern North American Society*. New Brunswick: Rutgers University Press.

Frankenberg, G. (1988) *AIDS-Bekämpfung im Rechtsstaat, Aufklärung–Zwang–Prävention*. Baden-Baden: Nomos.

Frankenberg, G. (1990) In the beginning of all the world was America: AIDS policy and law in West Germany, *New York University Journal of International Law and Politics*, 23, 5, 1079–109.

Freeman, R. (1992) Governing the voluntary sector response to AIDS: a comparative study of the UK and Germany, *Voluntas*, 3, 1, 29–47.

Garfield, S. (1994) *The End of Innocence: Britain in the Time of AIDS*. London: Faber.

Government of France (1987) *Circular letter DGS/1C no. 784 of 8 December 1987 concerning the health inspection of foreigners wishing to stay in France*. Paris: France.

Hall, P.A. and Lamont, M. (2009) *Successful Societies: How Institutions and Culture Affect Health*. Cambridge: Cambridge University Press.

Hamers, F., Devaux, I., Alix, J. and Nardone, A. (2006) HIV/AIDS in Europe: trends and EU-wide priorities, *European Surveillance* 11, 47, E061123.

Hepburn, E. (2008) The neglected nation: the CSU and the territorial cleavage in Bavarian party politics, *German Politics*, 17, 2, 184–202.

Hepburn, E. (2009) Regionalist party mobilisation on immigration, *West European Politics*, 32, 3, 514–35.

Ingleby, D. (1982) The social construction of mental illness. In Wright, P. and Treacher, A. (eds) *The Problem of Medical Knowledge*. Edinburgh: Edinburgh University Press.

Ingram, A. (2008) Domopolitics and disease: HIV/AIDS, immigration, and asylum in the UK, *Environment and Planning D: Society and Space*, 26, 5, 875–94.

Jenson, J. (2007) The European Union's citizenship regime. Creating norms and building practices, *Comparative European Politics*, 5, 1, 53–69.

Judt, T. (2001) Europe is one – until disaster strikes. 6 February. The New York Times. Available at http://www.nytimes.com/2001/02/06/opinion/europe-is-one-until-disaster-strikes.html?pagewanted=all&src=pm

Klaudt, K. (2000) The political causes and solutions of the current tuberculosis epidemic. In Whitman, J. (ed.) *The Politics of Emerging and Resurgent Infectious Diseases*. New York: St Martin's Press.

Klein, A. (2001) HIV/AIDS and Immigration: Final Report: Canadian HIV/AIDS Legal Network. Toronto: Canadian HIV/AIDS Legal Network. Available at http://www.aidslaw.ca/publications/interfaces/downloadFile.php?ref=853

Lazarus, J., Curth, N., Weait, M. and Matic, S. (2010) HIV-related restrictions on entry, residence and stay in the WHO European Region: a survey, *Journal of the International AIDS Society*, 13, 2. doi: 10.1186/1758-2652-13-2.

Lerner, B.H. (1997) From careless consumptives to recalcitrant patients: the historical construction of noncompliance, *Social Science & Medicine*, 45, 9, 1423–31.

Merry, S.E. (2006) Transnational human rights and local activism: mapping the middle, *American Anthropologist*, 108, 1, 38–51.

NAM (2010) *Dispersal of People Living with HIV*, aidsmap. London: NAM Publications.

Nolan, C.M. (1997) Editorial: nosocomial multidrug-resistant tuberculosis: global spread of the third epidemic, *Journal of Infectious Diseases*, 176, 3, 748–51.

Norredam, M., Mygind, A. and Krasnik, A. (2006) Access to health care for asylum seekers in the European Union—a comparative study of country policies, *European Journal of Public Health*, 16, 3, 285–9.

Pollak, M. (1990) AIDS in West Germany: coordinating policy in a federal system. In Misztal, B.A. and Moss, D. (eds) *Action on AIDS: National Policies in Comparative Perspective*. Westport, CT: Greenwood.

Raviglione, M.C. (2007) The new stop TB strategy and the global plan to stop TB, 2006–2015, *Bulletin of the World Health Organization*, 85, 5, 327–7.

Rose, A., Watson, J., Graham, C. and Nunn, A. *et al*. (2001) Tuberculosis at the end of the 20th century in England and Wales: results of a national survey in 1998, *Thorax*, 56, 3, 173–9.

Rosenberg, C.E. (1992) Framing disease: illness, society, and history. In Rosenberg, C.E. and Golden, J. (eds) *Framing Disease: Studies in Cultural History*. New Brunswick: Rutgers University Press.

Rosenberg, C.E. (2002) The tyranny of diagnosis: specific entities and individual experience, *Milbank Quarterly*, 80, 2, 237–60.

Shilts, R. (2007) *And the Band Played On: Politics, People, and the AIDS Epidemic*. New York: St Martin's Griffin.

Smith-Nonini, S. (2004) The cultural politics of institutional responses to resurgent tuberculosis epidemics. In Packard, R.M., Brown, P.J., Berkelman, R.L. and Frumkin, H. (eds) *Emerging Illnesses and Society: Negotiating the Public Health Agenda*. Baltimore and London: Johns Hopkins University Press.

Sontag, S. (1978) *Illness as Metaphor*. New York: Farrar, Strauss and Giroux.

Soysal, Y.N. (2001, 2004) Postnational citizenship: reconfiguring the familiar terrain. In Nash, K. and Scott, A. (eds) *The Blackwell Companion to Political Sociology*. Oxford: Blackwell.

Sutherland, C. (2001) Nation, Heimat, Vaterland: the reinvention of concepts by the Bavarian CSU, *German Politics*, 10, 3, 13–36.

UK Home Office, Border and Immigration Agency (2012) Migrant Tuberculosis Screening.

Wailoo, K. (1999) *Drawing Blood: Technology and Disease Identity in Twentieth-Century America*. Baltimore and London: Johns Hopkins University Press.

Walls, T. and Shingadia, D. (2007) The epidemiology of tuberculosis in Europe, *Archives of Disease in Childhood*, 92, 8, 726–9.

Weir, M. and Skocpol, T. (1985) State structures and the possibilities for 'Keynesian' responses to the Great Depression in Sweden, Britain, and the United States. In Evans, P., Rueschemeyer, D and Skocpol, T. (eds) *Bringing the State Back In*. New York: Cambridge University Press.

Welshman, J. (2006) Compulsion, localism, and pragmatism: the micro-politics of tuberculosis screening in the United Kingdom, 1950–1965, *Social History of Medicine*, 19, 2, 295–312.

Wiessner, P. and Lemmen, K. (2002) *Quick Reference – Travel and Residence Regulations for People with HIV and AIDS – Material for Counsellors in AIDS Service Organisations*. Berlin: Deutsche AIDS-Hilfe e.V.

World Health Organization (2008) *International Health Regulations (2005)* 2nd edn. Geneva: WHO.

8

The return of the city-state: Urban governance and the New York City H1N1 pandemic
Lily M. Hoffman

Introduction

For Weber (1986), a defining institutional feature of the city was as a unit of defence, a function taken over by the modern nation-state with its claims to exclusive jurisdiction within territorial boundaries. Commonly known as the Westphalian system of sovereign states (after the Treaty of Westphalia, 1648), this system of governance marked the weakening of local autonomy and the assignment of Weber's classic definition of the city to the dustbin of history. However, the emergence of supranational organisations, and non-state actors with claims to authority, in an interdependent, globalised world has generated discussion of a *post*-Westphalian order[1] and the re-assessment of governance issues.

Urban theorists have proposed that cities are both facing new demands within a restructuring global economy and experiencing a downward drift of authority from the national level. Global cities theory (Brenner and Keil 2006, Friedmann 1986, Sassen 1991) asserts that cities have taken on (economic) command and control functions within global networks, variously described in terms of nodes, as a space of flows (Castells 1996) and as a porous spatial order (Taylor and Derudder 2004). Studies of new institutional capacity and governance have found that restructuring has given localities more initiative, particularly in regard to economic development (Brenner 2004, Harvey 1989).

Critical of an overemphasis on economic functions, others have revived the Weberian model, with its concern for socio-political as well as economic factors. The rise of supranational organisations, such as the European Union, is seen to have been accompanied by greater self-direction and policy initiative for the enlarged city or metropolitan region (Bagnasco and Le Gales 2000, Kazepov 2004). Haussermann and Haila (2004: 7) suggest the Weberian city might function as 'a new research paradigm', raising questions about the conditions that create opportunities for cities to become political actors and envisioning a more constructivist model of governance. Borraz and Le Galès (2010: 6) suggest that the city has become a 'locus of risk' (protests, crime, disease) which can 'contribute to a redefinition of boundaries between state and different levels of government'.

The re-emergence of infectious disease, alongside globalisation, has provoked security concerns in the face of heightened vulnerability. Although cities have historically been the unit of planning and response to disease, in the post-Westphalian era, most attention has

Pandemics and Emerging Infectious Diseases: The Sociological Agenda, First Edition. Edited by Robert Dingwall, Lily M. Hoffman and Karen Staniland. Chapters © 2013 The Authors. Book Compilation © 2013 Foundation for the Sociology of Health & Illness / John Wiley & Sons Ltd.

been directed at the global nature of the threat and the relationship between nation-states and the supranational World Health Organization (WHO). Fidler (2003: 485) identifies a new non-state-centric health governance template. He argues that, during the 2003 out-break of acute respiratory syndrome (SARS) (the 'first post-Westphalian Pathogen'), the WHO gained a significant degree of technical control over global health.[2] But Fidler also notes that the recognition of infectious disease as a national security threat raises the possibility of returning to a state-centric model. Critics of the global health governance thesis acknowledge the shift, but note the continuing importance of the nation-state (Ricci 2010).

Working on SARS within the post-Westphalian framework, Ali and Keil link infectious disease to both global cities theory (2006) and the urban governance literature (Keil and Ali 2007). In their study of Toronto during the 2003 SARS epidemic, they describe how city and provincial public health officials became political actors, lobbying the WHO to rescind a travel advisory (Keil and Ali 2007). They also note the relative ineffectiveness of Canadian national health governance and find, in the aftermath, a tendency for more resources and authority to accrue to subnational levels (Ali and Keil 2008). Cities and metropolitan regions are also receiving more attention from health policymakers. In October 2008, for example, the WHO organised a technical consultation on threats to cities from emerging infectious disease in Lyons, France (WHO 2008).

Methods and map

The case of New York City (NYC) and the 2009 H1N1 pandemic sheds further light on the evolving nature of health governance in relation to contemporary outbreaks of infec-tious disease. It is particularly interesting because, after the terrorist attacks on September 11 2001 ('9/11'), the USA reframed and institutionalised infectious disease as a national security risk, as hypothesised by Fidler (2003). Although the WHO triggered the alert levels, the key actors were city and national governments. This study examines the outcomes of their interaction.

Did NYC retain control over health governance and if so, what made this possible? Several methods have been used to address these questions.

First, to present the event in its institutional context I have used interviews, online and documentary analysis. Ten semi-structured interviews were conducted with members of local and national public health organisations involved in decision-making. Online and media analysis were used to construct a timeline of events. During the outbreak, the websites of NYC Department of Health and Mental Health (DOHMH), the Centers for Disease Control and Prevention (CDC) and other health organisations were monitored. Scientific, medical and legal literature pertaining to H1N1, the 2009 H1N1 pandemic and pandemic planning was reviewed.

Second, all-hazards pandemic planning and its impact were documented through analy-sis of federal and state legislation, policy statements, congressional reports and interviews. In Spring 2009 I made an informal survey of internet-disseminated predictions of the H1N1 trajectory in the USA. The impact of the event was also evaluated through a post-hoc examination of 'lessons learned', based on hearings and published reports through Fall 2011.

In the following sections, I first discuss the organisational and ideological context for NYC pandemic planning; then examine how H1N1 actually played out during Spring and Fall 2009. As noted, the post-9/11 national security regime, which includes planning for the emergence of infectious disease, is central to this analysis. What was its impact on NYC's pandemic response? What did it mean in terms of health governance?

The organisational and ideological context for pandemic planning

NYC as a unit of health policy and planning
The US's constitutional division of functions between state and federal government gives legal jurisdiction over citizens' health to the states. This means that all states have health departments, but not all counties and cities. Cities like NYC, with over 8.2 million residents, have large health departments with an expansive range of activities and a complex set of institutional partners. With over 6,000 employees and a budget of $1.6 billion, the DOHMH is one of the world's largest public health agencies. It interacts with a large public and private health sector which includes a public hospital system, several 'medical empires', one of six national centers for public health preparedness, major corporate headquarters and the United Nations. Finally, the department oversees public health nurses in over 1900 schools and healthcare for 13,000 prisoners.

The public health system is both vertical and horizontal, with localities positioned at one end of a scale that goes through state and national levels to supranational organisations like the WHO. At the national level, jurisdiction is fragmented: eight agencies, including the US Department of Health and Human Services (HHS) and several offices, carry out public health functions as well as the CDC, a branch of HHS. States, which have principal authority over public health, typically delegate some authority to localities; some of which, like NYC, essentially have 'home rule' over public health (Lister 2005: 11).

The post-9/11 environment for pandemic planning: All-hazards and emergency preparedness

> Many in the medical community turned to us during the events of September 11, 2001 and their aftermath for up-to-date information on anthrax, air quality, and other challenging problems. (Dr Thomas R. Frieden, former Commissioner, NYC DOHMH 2003)

During the post-cold war threat climate commonly referred to as '9/11', infectious disease was redefined as a national security matter (HSC 2005). In addition to their traditional responsibilities for infectious disease and food-borne illnesses, public health departments found their agenda expanded to encompass preparation for a wide range of other emergencies – an 'all-hazards' approach that included blast injuries, natural disasters and radiological and chemical events, along with bioterrorism (Levi *et al.* 2009: 7, US Government Pandemic and All-Hazards Preparedness Act [PAHPA] 2006). One consequence is that the protocols and rhetoric of emergency preparedness and risk management have permeated all facets of public health: research, training, methods and practice.

Although concern with potential chemical and bioterrorism threats preceded 9/11 with such incidents as the Sarin attack in Japan, anthrax threats and novel viruses such as West Nile, the impetus for integrating emergency management and pandemic planning became compelling after 9/11 with a sharp increase in funding and research grants.[3] The rationale was the concept of *dual-use*: that 'the strong infrastructure needed to respond to natural disease threats will also improve the response to the threat of terrorism' (Lister 2005: 1). Public health officials, who faced the re-emergence of infectious disease with declining support for public health, found a strategic alignment with emergency preparedness to be a godsend. In terms of policy, dual-use offered a way to move beyond planning for specific scenarios to a more generic assessment of threats and vulnerabilities and the possibility of establishing priorities (Lister 2005: 2, 21).

As institutionalised in federal legislation and directives, the all-hazards approach to emergency preparedness has the following organisational and methodological characteristics:

- All-hazards preparedness introduced a new layer of bureaucracy with public health responsibilities. The Homeland Security Act (2002) established the Department of Homeland Security (DHS) and its local branch, the Office of Emergency Management (OEM). The 2006 Pandemic and All-Hazards Preparedness Act (PAPHA) brought emergency preparedness planning directly into the HHS (US Government PAHPA 2006). Since 2002, a series of laws and operational directives have sought, somewhat unsuccessfully, to clarify organisational structures and define relations between the DHS and the HHS.
- The all-hazards approach represents a concerted effort to create standardised models for detection and response and to bring states and localities into compliance with these standards. An example is the National Incident Management System (NIMS), a prerequisite for receiving federal emergency preparedness grants, developed by DHS in 2004. The NIMS requires the establishment of a Citywide Incident Management System (CIMS), which identifies and coordinates leadership and support for emergencies through a Citywide Incident Command Structure. Similar templates include the CDC-sponsored Model State Public Health Act (Centers for Law and the Public's Health 2003).
- Emergency preparedness has promoted medical surveillance technology or medical informatics by applying traditional tools of public health (syndromic surveillance, case tracking) to detect bioterrorism and other events and by relabelling epidemiologists as 'disease detectives' (HSS 2002).
- Public health has turned to statistical analysis and computer modelling to deal with unpredictability. The CDC created a Preparedness Modeling Unit in 2008, to apply probabilistic statistics to both spread and response issues, making infectious disease management a 'predictive science' (Rosenfeld 2008: 4). The ultimate goal is to develop software models, train local health departments to plug in data and make decisions on the basis of the models. Respondents in a CDC-sponsored survey of health departments (including NYC) raised concerns about the use of models, noting that their utility depended on their assumptions. They also raised questions of scalability, reliability and competent staffing. Interestingly, computer modelling was valued as a political tool, such as in convincing local officials to close schools (Rosenfeld 2008: 13–14). Adopting this approach, the WHO convened an informal network in 2009 to apply mathematical modelling to the H1N1 pandemic (Van Kerkhove *et al.* 2010).
- Worst-case scenarios have been widely adopted: Alessandro Vespignani, an expert in computer based epidemic modelling, observed 'we are always working in a worst-case scenario setting' (Indiana University 2009). My Spring 2009 survey of Internet disseminated predictions, found that the most common computer simulations – with video and podcast – were 'worst-case'.
- Another strategy associated with unpredictable events is the preparedness exercise. A well-known example is Atlantic Storm (2005), a bioterrorism exercise that convened a summit of transatlantic leaders for eight hours to respond to a smallpox attack. NYC's 2006 Pandemic Preparedness Plan noted that DOHMH had 'engaged in extensive preparedness efforts – over 50 tabletop and full-scale exercises in the past five years' (New York City Department of Health and Mental Hygiene [NYC DOHMH] 2006: 3).
- The all-hazards approach has colonised public health with a law-enforcement perspective. A 2008 White Paper by the American Civil Liberties Union (ACLU) argued that,

after 9/11, the Bush Administration's all–hazards approach encouraged 'overreaction', leading to the use of coercive strategies such as forced examinations, containment and criminal sanctions (Annas *et al.* 2008). One example is the CDC's Model State Public Health Act, drafted at the request of the Bush administration (Centers for Law and the Public's Health 2003). The act 'provided state officials with extensive, unchecked powers to curtail individual autonomy in the face of an emergency, including the power to compel vaccination, testing, treatment, and isolation' (Simoncelli 2009: 7). Described as a 'mini-Patriot Act', it became the model for federal and state emergency preparedness planning including New York State (Annas *et al.* 2008). The ACLU also noted that the law enforcement model shifted attention from community measures such as education, treatment and prevention to individuals (Annas *et al.* 2008). Critics have distinguished this 'neoliberal' focus from traditional public health activities (Petersen and Lupton 1996).

Rescaling up or down?
The all-hazards approach reflects the standardisation and centralisation of public health emergency preparedness activities under a national governance rubric. Some felt that 9/11 made the case for a stronger national role. Faced with a decentralised public health system, whose basic authority resided at the state level and a fragmented healthcare system, predominately in private hands (Lister and Gottran 2007: 1), Congress made public health an issue of national security, establishing federal leadership roles and channelling federal funds to states and localities.

At the same time, 9/11 also underlined the essentially local nature of threat and the need to prepare first responders. No-one looked back to the 1976 Swine Flu Program – a national vaccination campaign – as a model; it was considered a disaster (Neustadt *et al.* 1978). Moreover, it was recognised that localities differed in needs and resources: while public health had to be strengthened at state and local level, one size did not fit all. 9/11 thus foregrounded existing tensions between federal initiatives and state and locality control.

The event: H1N1 in NYC – spring and fall 2009

H1N1, a new variant of influenza A and the first global pandemic since the 1968 Hong Kong flu, had its first major US outbreak in NYC in late April 2009. Traced to students returning from a spring break in Mexico City, where a widespread outbreak had occurred, the onset was dramatic, with the school acting as a transmission point. Within a few days, hundreds of children were sick and public concern became frenzied (Lessler *et al.* 2009).

Given the lack of information about the new influenza strain, the reported severity of the Mexico City outbreak and the rising WHO alert (level 5 of 6 on 29 April), DOHMH launched a pandemic response. This activated the agency-wide incident command system (ICS), which assigned all employees to on-call teams, shifting from a 'routine' to an 'enhanced' surveillance system. During the Spring, the ICS was activated twice for enhanced surveillance, operating seven days a week from 9 A.M. to 9 P.M to monitor the pandemic and use the results to guide response (Balter *et al.* 2010). During the first ICS activation (25 April–8 May), there were few severe cases (only 15 hospitalisations). Most were linked to the school influenza outbreak. By the end of the second ICS activation (19 May–7 July) there were over 900 hospitalised cases. An estimated 750,000 to one million people – about 10 per cent of NYC's population – had H1N1 during Spring 2009 and there were 930 hospitalisations with 54 deaths (Chan and Foderaro 2009).

The DOHMH initially used school closings as a mitigation tactic. This followed NYC's pandemic preparedness plan, as well as CDC guidance, which initially recommended that schools with at least one confirmed case immediately close for up to two weeks (Klaiman *et al.* 2011). Between April and mid-June 60 schools were closed for no more than five days, at first to limit transmission and, later, to protect those more vulnerable (Department of Education 2009). By early July the outbreak had died down. Public health officials, thinking historically of the trajectory of flu epidemics – their affinity for cooler weather and the virus's propensity to mutate – expected a return in the Fall, probably in a more severe form.

The outbreak raised questions about NYC's response and provoked a policy review. In early June a City Council committee met key actors to review the spring experience and assess preparations for the Fall. The lead NYC agencies – DOHMH and OEM – were questioned by Council members. There was little praise for NYC's handling of the outbreak from the media, other city agencies or the public. Questions were raised regarding school policy – the lack of a clear set of criteria, the availability of medical services, the adequacy of communications and the lack of transparency regarding mortality, morbidity and school statistics (NYC City Council Committee on Health, Governmental Operations and Public Safety 2009). One general criticism was an overemphasis on maintaining public order.

Fall 2009

Having decided that the second H1N1 wave would be more moderate and with a better idea of the groups at risk, Health Commissioner Dr Thomas Farley and Mayor Bloomberg announced a Fall plan that was 'equal parts infection control and panic control' (Chan and Foderaro 2009). In three pages, DOHMH laid out its strategy: first and foremost, an 'open school' policy. Schools would close only as a last resort and would stress basic prevention. School children would receive free vaccinations (once available); health clinics would relieve hospitals; daily statistics would be posted on the web; NYC would establish a call centre and a volunteer corps, and would maintain emergency stockpiles of antivirals (NYC DOHMH 2009).

Central to NYC's Fall pandemic plan was the assessment of the virus. By Fall 2009 DOHMH had enough data to re-evaluate the risk to individuals and found it to be much lower than originally expected. H1N1 was milder than seasonal flu and vaccines would soon be available. With severity downgraded, DOHMH retreated from disruptive measures such as school closings and called for less resource-intensive surveillance. The emphasis was placed on preventative measures at school, the workplace and the home (Farley 2009). The plan also emphasised public communication of up-to-the minute information about the virus.

NYC garnered praise for its moderate approach to H1N1 in Fall 2009, as being more evidence based than the response in Mexico City. Events also conspired for a happy ending: the Fall recurrence was very mild. Although highly transmissible in children, the virus was rarely lethal, did not mutate and was susceptible to drugs.

All-hazards emergency preparedness and pandemic response

Our observations about the fit between all-hazards and DOHMH'S efforts during the 2009 pandemic follow.

Bureaucratic interface citywide

Despite overlapping functions between competing agencies, CIMS worked as planned to divide responsibilities, identify a leadership structure and, on the whole, prevent jurisdictional infighting. In a public health emergency, CIMS identifies the lead agency as the Department of Health, which then activates its own ICS and receives support from the OEM, the police, fire and other city entities. During the crisis, the DOHMH and OEM held daily conference calls with City Hall, the Department of Education, the Department of Corrections, the Health and Hospitals Corporation and other agencies. Despite the potential competition over leadership, OEM took a secondary role, providing logistical support and coordination and enabling DOHMH to concentrate on the outbreak. However, given that the H1N1 pandemic was a clear-cut public health issue, unlike, for example, bioterrorism, the organisational outcome would likely have been the same in this case without the CIMS protocol.

Resources and capacity
Because all-hazards includes a variety of dangers alongside pandemic flu, it provided greater support to the public health department. Extra funding for emergencies enabled DOHMH to activate enhanced surveillance and epidemiology, improved public health laboratories and supported a Bureau of Emergency Management within DOHMH. DOHMH was also included in emergency preparation and training exercises. Additionally, all-hazards included funding for each NYC hospital to create its own ICS which enhanced DOHMH's overall surveillance capacity. According to members of the NYC 2009 H1N1 flu investigation team, 'surveillance data were critical in guiding the DOHMH response' (Balter *et al.* 2010: 1259).

One could argue that, if emergency preparedness funding only went to those agencies we typically think of as first responders, such as the police, fire or the OEM, the public health component of planning might be overlooked. As it is, the renewed importance of large-scale emergencies and their inclusion within public health has made the health department an increasingly important function in urban policy and planning.

Models, projections, worst-case scenarios
At the same time, the reframing and institutionalisation of infectious disease within all-hazards emergency preparedness has given rise to assumptions and strategies that may be unrealistic and potentially at odds with effective pandemic response.

During the Spring/Fall H1N1 outbreak, NYC's pandemic preparedness plan did not provide accurate guidance to decision-makers. Relying on models based upon a number of assumptions about incidence and severity and about vaccines and antiviral drugs, DOHMH officials found their plan overestimated the severity of the threat: it assumed 30 per cent of the population would become infected; 11 per cent of those infected would be hospitalised and 2.1 per cent of the infected would die (NYC DOHMH 2006). In reality this was a mild pandemic and NYC estimated that only 10–12 per cent of New Yorkers were infected during the Spring, only 0.1 per cent of those infected were hospitalised and deaths accounted for only 0.007 per cent of those hospitalised (Chan and Foderaro 2009). A response based on guidelines that differ widely from reality can lead to overreaction, an issue raised in regard to the spring school closings as well as to the New York State Department of Health's decision to vaccinate all state health workers.

School closing policy
In the initial stage, when so little was known about the virus, DOHMH closed schools in which there were either confirmed cases of H1N1 or unusually high levels of flu-like symptoms. By the end of May, with surveillance data showing that spread occurred outside the schools, it had become clear that closing schools was ineffective in containing the virus. The NYC Fall 2009 plans were more moderate than in Spring 2009: significantly more so than

other forecasts, including the 'plausible' baseline scenario for H1N1's return from the President's Council of Advisors on Science and Technology (PCAST), which posited that 30–50 per cent of the US population could become infected (in NYC that would have been 2–4 million people), with 30,000 to 90,000 deaths (PCAST 2009). It was primarily the reduction of uncertainty through greater scientific knowledge that led to NYC's updated school closing policy.

Mandatory vaccination and civil rights
The NY State Department of Health's decision to impose mandatory vaccination on all state health workers sharply contrasts with NYC's Fall plan. Drawing on powers conferred by the state's emergency health powers legislation, New York was the *only* state to require mandatory vaccinations and did so when it was already known that H1N1 was much less dangerous than had originally been thought. The state quickly found itself up against strong criticism from labour unions and the New York Civil Liberties Union on the grounds that the rule 'could result in the punishment and even dismissal of workers who refuse, whether for religious, cultural or other reasons, to be vaccinated' (Hartocollis 2009). A lawsuit led to a restraining order and State Governor Patterson suspended the law in October (Simoncelli 2009).

The media were also captive to a worst-case scenario. Rather than explaining that plans were based on an extreme projection and that much about the virus was unknown, the media tended to present a dramatic, albeit simplified, story. The public health establishment was similarly criticised for failing to clarify whether their recommendations were based on models or real data and for failing to explain how they balanced control of infection with the need to maintain daily life (Wenzel 2010). In the aftermath, most criticism for overreaction has been directed at the WHO for raising the threat level even though it was evident that the virus was milder than seasonal flu. The WHO – and global governance in general – have also been criticised by an international review panel on H1N1 influenza for its '"needlessly complex" definition of pandemic, with six levels of alert, based on the virus's geographical spread, not its severity' (McNeil 2011). The danger of rote use of plans based on worst-case scenarios is the loss of credibility. Commenting on New York State's attempt to impose mandatory vaccination, CDC Director and former head of NYC's DOHMH, Dr Thomas Frieden stated, 'this is just not the right flu season to take this on' (Hartocollis and Chan 2009).

The problem of initial response
We have noted that NYC's pandemic preparedness plan was based on unrealistic assumptions about severity. Although DOHMH went on to use its epidemiological and surveillance capacity to gather its own data and revised its Fall policy accordingly, this does not solve the problem of what to do at the start. Despite attempts to reduce uncertainty by calculating the probability of a given risk, some decisions may remain stubbornly elusive. Discussing the management of uncertainty related to the H1N1 virus, an article in the *New England Journal of Medicine* argues that the key issue at the start is how to predict 'severity' with any degree of confidence. Estimates suffer from two sources of uncertainty: overestimation of severe cases (because mild cases are not counted) and a downward bias because there is a delay between onset and death (Lipsitch *et al.* 2009). Given the idiosyncratic nature of viruses, the authors are not optimistic about reducing such uncertainty. One might also note that, despite advanced technology-based surveillance systems such as Bio Watch and Biosurveillance, the first notice of the NYC outbreak came from an 'alert clinician', a school nurse (Bell *et al.* 2009: 311).

Within the medical community, some have argued that public health officials need to be more transparent about what *they do not know* about a given virus (Wenzel 2010). Similar concerns have been raised in regard to specific policies. Reviewing national school closures during the 2009 H1N1 pandemic, Klaiman *et al.* (2011) argue that too little is known about the effect of containment strategies, such as school closings, on the spread, morbidity and mortality of flu.

In answer to the question of the impact of the federally mandated all-hazards approach on NYC's response to the 2009 H1N1 pandemic, the results are mixed. Additional funding and preparatory exercises added resources and skills and put the issue of emergency preparation at the top of DOHMH's agenda. The federally mandated protocols reaffirmed the department's centrality and decision-making authority in the pandemic, although this probably would have been the case in their absence. At the same time, the standardised, federally mandated, model-driven approach did not translate well into an appropriate local response; the basic assumptions of 'all-hazards' planning did not match the reality of a mild pandemic. Modelling may have its limitations, particularly in the initial stages and it remains to be seen how far it fits with an evidence-based approach.

The law enforcement approach also gave rise to concerns about civil liberties as in the attempt to mandate vaccination for New York State health workers or in the debate about school closings. As noted above, NYC's more moderate approach in Fall 2009 shifted the focus from 'social' to 'individual' responsibility. Although criticised by some as a neoliberal revision of public health, this means something different in the USA than in Canada or the UK. Countries with some form of universal health service seem more accepting of social approaches. In the USA, social strategies such as school closings, disease testing or mandated vaccination tend to be more negatively viewed as forms of social control.

Implications for health governance

In the USA, the resurgence of infectious disease has been met by the assertion of state authority. Reframed and institutionalised as a matter of national security, pandemic planning and response operates within an all-hazards emergency preparedness framework. What did this mean in terms of actual health governance? During the NYC H1N1 pandemic, the reality was local control with DOHMH the effective unit of decision-making and action.

One can explain this outcome through a reading of the agency/structure debate that sees the two as mutually constitutive (Giddens 1984). As institutionalised, the rhetoric and protocols of all-hazards emergency preparedness propelled NYC into action as a prepared first responder. The lack of fit between the federally mandated framework with its worst-case scenarios and the mild H1N1 outbreak provided the opportunity for NYC to seize the initiative by developing its own plans for the return of H1N1 in Fall 2009, based on its own reading of the evidence.

At the same time, agent-specific characteristics – the size, resource level and experience of DOHMH, its surveillance capacity, the expertise of local public health officials, as well as their close working relationship with CDC, were all crucially important. This meant that with minimal back-up, DOHMH was able to follow their plan as warranted and improvise more realistic solutions as needed. Thus a combination of structurally induced opportunity and actor specific strengths facilitated effective local governance. Not all local public health departments would have been able to seize the policy initiative and act as effectively; however several other large US cities and metropolitan areas have health departments similar to New York's.

Looking at 'lessons learned' from the 2009 NYC H1N1 pandemic gives us additional insight into the governance issue. A review of reports and studies published up to Fall 2011 finds that they emphasise the importance of on-the-scene surveillance and evaluation, flexibility and adaptability, deference to local knowledge and authority and evidence-based policy.[4] Although revised models may solve some of the specific problems encountered in NYC, they will not necessarily change the overall conclusion, which emphasises local initiative and decision-making and the need for adequate resources for first responders. Moreover, because it is not clear that a technical fix can eliminate uncertainty, response may remain dependent on the locality and thus on actor-specific characteristics – the mix of local expertise and resource capacity – and therefore remain unevenly distributed spatially.

In underlining the importance of the locality as a first line of defence for threats of infectious disease and linking this function to policy initiative in regard to health governance, this study illustrates the continuing relevance of Weber's insight into the institutional structure of the city. Although NYC may be particularly qualified to exhibit autonomy regarding security functions and although various political, economic and cultural factors may affect the ability of other localities to act in a similar fashion, to the extent that localities face threats to their security, they will need to defend themselves. To do so effectively, they need *more* rather than less autonomy. Along these lines, health policy should pay more attention to cities and metropolitan areas as agents of health governance; urbanists should note that the rescaling of governance can be a function of defence or security as well as economic needs.

Acknowledgements

I wish to thank Michael Grant for his research assistance and the Charles B. Rangel Center at CCNY/CUNY for supporting a graduate assistant. An earlier version of this chapter was presented at the International Sociological Meetings in Goteborg Sweden, July 2010. I also wish to thank the anonymous reviewers at the *Sociology of Health and Illness* for their perceptive comments.

Notes

1 Supra-state organizations (such as the European Union) and non-state actors (such as Human Rights Watch, the Organization of the Petroleum Exporting Countries, Al Qaida) are among the challenges that have contributed to this reformulation of international relations.
2 The WHO has become increasingly influential over the past 30 years, setting global standards including criteria for pandemics and monitoring surveillance (Swendiman and Jones 2009: 7).
3 From 2002 to 2010 Congress gave $11.4 billion in grants to states to build public health and medical capacity in preparation for health-related threats (Lister 2011, Figures 1 and 2: 6, 8).
4 Among others: Balter *et al.* (2010), Bell *et al.* (2009), Farley (2009), Klaiman *et al.* (2011), Levi *et al.* (2009), Lister (2011), McKenna (2009), Schnirring (2011), Schuchat *et al.* (2011), Simoncelli (2009), PCAST (2009), Steinhardt (2009), Swendiman and Jones (2009), US Department of Education (2009).

References

Ali, S.H. and Keil, R. (2006) Global cities and the spread of infectious disease: the case of severe acute respiratory syndrome (SARS) in Toronto, Canada, *Urban Studies*, 43, 3, 491–509.

Ali, S.H. and Keil, R. (2008) SARS and the restructuring of health governance in Toronto. In Ali, S.H. and Keil, R. (eds) *Networked Disease: Emerging Infections in the Global City*. Malden: Wiley-Blackwell.

Annas, G., Mariner, W. and Parmet, W. (2008) *Pandemic Preparedness: the Need for a Public Health – Not a Law Enforcement/National Security – Approach*. American Civil Liberties Union, available at http://www.aclu.org/pdfs/privacy/pemic_report.pdf (accessed 21 April 2012).

Bagnasco, A. and Le Gales, P. (eds) (2000) *Cities in Contemporary Europe*. Cambridge: Cambridge University Press.

Balter, S., Gupta, L., Lim, S., Fu, J., *et al.* (2010) Pandemic (H1N1) 2009 surveillance for severe illness and response, April–July 2009, *Emerging Infectious Diseases*, 16, 10, available at http://wwwnc.cdc.gov/eid/article/16/8/09-1847_article.htm (accessed 21 April 2012).

Bell, D., Weisfuse, I., Hernandez-Avila, I., del Rio, C., *et al.* (2009) Pandemic influenza as 21 century urban public health crisis, *Emerging Infectious Diseases*, 15, 12, 1963–9.

Borraz, O. and Le Galès, P. (2010) *Urban Governance in Europe: the Government of What?* Metropoles, 7, available at http://metropoles.revues.org/4297 (accessed 21 April 2012).

Brenner, N. (2004) *New State Spaces*. New York: Oxford.

Brenner, N. and Keil, R. (eds) (2006) *The Global Cities Reader*. New York: Routledge.

Castells, M. (1996) *The Rise of the Network Society*. Oxford: Blackwell.

Centers for Law and the Public's Health (2003) The Turning Point Model State Public Health Act. Washington, D.C., available at http://www.hss.state.ak.us/dph/improving/turningpoint/MSPHA.htm (accessed 1 May 2012).

Chan, S. and Foderaro, I. (2009) This time, city says it's ready for swine flu. *The New York Times*, 2 September.

Farley, T. (2009) Testimony before Committee on Homeland Security, U.S. House of Representatives. *Beyond Readiness: An Examination of the Current Status and Future Outlook of the National Response to Pandemic Influenza*. Washington, 29 July, available at http://hsc-democrats.house.gov/hearings/index.asp?ID=209 (accessed 21 April 2012).

Fidler, D. (2003) SARS: Political pathology of the first post-Westphalian pathogen, *Journal of Law, Medicine and Ethics*, 31, 4, 485–505.

Frieden, T. (2003) *Letter to New Members of the NYC Medical Community*, 3 June, available at http://www.nyc.gov/html/doh/downloads/pdf/public/newhealthcare.pdf (accessed 21 April 2012).

Friedmann, J. (1986) The world city hypothesis, *Development and Change*, 17, 1, 69–84.

Giddens, A. (1984) *The Constitution of Society*. Berkeley: University of California Press.

Hartocollis, A. (2009) Mandatory flu vaccination for N.Y. health workers is criticized, *The New York Times*, 14 October.

Hartocollis, A. and Chan, S. (2009) Flu vaccine requirement for health workers is lifted, *The New York Times*, 23 October.

Harvey, D. (1989) From managerialism to entrepreneurialism: the transformation of urban governance in late capitalism, *Geografiska Annaler*, 71B, 1, 3–17.

Haussermann, H. and Haila, A. (2004) The European city: a conceptual framework and normative project. In Kazepov, Y. (ed.) *Cities of Europe*. Oxford: Blackwell.

Indiana University (2009) *Swine Flu: Statistical Model Predicts 1,000 Cases In U.S. Within Three Weeks, ScienceDaily*, 29 April, available at http://www.sciencedaily.com/releases/2009/04/090429171015.htm (accessed 21 April 2012).

Kazepov, Y. (ed.) (2004) *Cities of Europe*. Oxford: Blackwell.

Keil, R. and Ali, S. (2007) Governing the sick city: urban governance in the age of emerging infectious disease, *Antipode* 39, 5, 846–73.

Klaiman, T., Kraemer, J. and Stoto, M. (2011) Variability in school closure decisions in response to 2009 H1N1, *BMC Public Health*, 11, 73, available at http://www.biomedcentral.com/1471-2458/11/73/abstract (accessed 21 April 2012).

Lessler, J., Reich, N.J., Cummings, D.A.T. and the New York City Department of Health and Mental Hygiene Swine Influenza Investigation Team (2009) Outbreak of 2009 pandemic influenza A (H1N1) at a New York City school, *New England Journal of Medicine*, 361, 27, 2628–36.

Levi, J., Vinter, S. and Segal, L. (2009) Ready or Not? Protecting the Public's Health from Diseases, Disasters, and Bioterrorism. Trust for America's Health (TFAH) and the Robert Wood Johnson Foundation, available at http://healthyamericans.org/reports/bioterror09/pdf/TFAHReadyorNot 200906.pdf (accessed 21 April 2012).

Lipsitch, M., Riley, S., Cauchemez, S., Ghani, A., *et al.* (2009) Managing and reducing uncertainty in an emerging influenza pandemic, *New England Journal of Medicine*, 361, 112–15.

Lister, S. (2005) *An Overview of the U.S. Public Health System in the Context of Emergency Preparedness.* Congressional Research Service (CRS Report RL31719). Washington: CRS.

Lister, S (2011) *Public Health and Medical Emergency Management: Issues in the 112 Congress.* Congressional Research Service (CRS Report R41646). Washington: CRS.

Lister, S. and Gottran, F. (2007) *The Pandemic and All-Hazards Preparedness Act (P.L. 109–417): Provisions and Changes to Preexisting Law.* Congressional Research Service (CRS Report RL33589). Washington: CRS.

McKenna, M. (2009) *CDC Advises Against Closing Schools During H1N1 Outbreaks*, available at http://www.cidrap.umn.edu/cidrap/content/influenza/panflu/news/aug0709schools3.html (accessed 21 April 2012).

McNeil D. Jr (2011) Response of W.H.O. to swine flu is criticized, *The New York Times*, 10 March.

Neustadt, R., Fineberg, H. and Califano, J. Jr. (1978) *The Swine Flu Affair: Decision-Making on a Slippery Disease.* Washington: U.S. Department of Health, Education and Welfare.

New York City Council Committee on Health, Governmental Operations and Public Safety (2009) *New York City's Response to H1N1 and Assessing Influenza Preparedness*, 11 June, available at http://legistar.council.nyc.gov/MeetingDetail.aspx?ID=76707&GUID=9B92BBCD-BAD7-4EBA-9BFC-FAE4A4DADE1B&Search= (accessed 21 April 2012).

New York City Department of Health and Mental Hygiene (NYC DOHMH) (2006) *Pandemic Influenza Preparedness and Response Plan*, available at http://www.nyc.gov/html/doh/downloads/pdf/cd/cd-panflu-plan.pdf (accessed 21 April 2012).

NYC DOHMH (2009) Health Department and Department of Education Announce Open-School Policy and a School-based Vaccination Initiative for the Fall/Winter Influenza Season. 1 September, available at http://www.nyc.gov/html/doh/html/pr2009/prj60-09.shtml (accessed 21 April 2012).

Petersen, A. and Lupton, D. (1996) *The New Public Health: Health and Self in the Age of Risk.* London: Sage.

President's Council of Advisors on Science and Technology (PCAST) (2009) *Report to President on U.S. Preparations for 2009-H1N1 Influenza.* Washington: Executive Office of the President, 7 August.

Ricci, J. (2009) H1N1 returns, again: the globalization, re-conceptualization and vaccination of 'swine flu', *Global Health Governance*, 3, 2.

Rosenfeld, L. (2008) A multi-state needs assessment consultation with state and local health officials concerning use of computer modeling for preparedness activities, *Journal of Public Health Management and Practice*, 15, 2, 96–104.

Sassen, S. (1991) *The Global City.* Princeton: Princeton University Press.

Schnirring, L. (2011) *UK Proposes More Flexible Pandemic Plan*, available at http://www.cidrap.umn.edu/cidrap/content/influenza/panflu/news/mar2211panplan.html (accessed 21 April 2012).

Schuchat, B., Bell, P. and Redd, S.C. (2011) The science behind preparing and responding to pandemic influenza: the lessons and limits of science, *Clinical Infectious Diseases*, 52 (suppl 1): S8–12.

Simoncelli, T. (2009) *Maintaining Civil Liberties Protections in Response to the H1N1 Flu.* American Civil Liberties Union (ACLU), available at http://www.aclu.org/files/assets/H1N1_Report_FINAL.pdf (accessed 21 April 2012).

Steinhardt, B. (2009) *Influenza Pandemic: Gaps in Pandemic Planning and Preparedness Need to Be Addressed.* U.S. GOA-09–909T, GOA Testimony before Committee on Homeland Security, Washington: House of Representatives.

Swendiman, K. and Jones, N. (2009) *The 2009 Influenza Pandemic: Selected Legal Issues.* Washington: Congressional Research Service (CRS Report R40560) 29 October.

Taylor, P.J. and Derudder, B. (2004) Porous Europe: European cities in global urban arenas, *Tidjschrift voor Economische en Sociale Geografie*, 95, 5, 527–38.

US Department of Education (2009) *Lessons Learned from School Crises and Emergencies*. 4:1, June, available at http://rems.ed.gov/docs/LL_Vol4Issue1.pdf (accessed 21 April 2012).

US Department of Health and Human Services (HHS) (2002) *Fiscal Year 2003 Budget in Brief*, available at http://archive.hhs.gov/budget/docbudgetarchive.htm#FY03 (accessed 21 April 2012).

US Government (2002) Homeland Security Act. Public Law 107–296. Washington D.C., available at: http://www.dhs.gov/xlibrary/assets/hr_5005_enr.pdf (accessed 1 May 2012)

US Government (2006) Pandemic and All-Hazards Preparedness Act [PAHPA]. Public Law 109–417. Washington, available at http://www.flu.gov/planning-preparedness/federal/pandemic-influenza.pdf (accessed 1 May 2012)

US Homeland Security Council (2005) *National Strategy for Pandemic Influenza*. Washington, available at http://www.flu.gov/planning-preparedness/federal/pandemic-influenza.pdf (accessed 21 April 2012).

Van Kerkhove, M., Asikainen, T., Becker, N., Bjorge, S., *et al.* (2010) Studies needed to address public health challenges of the 2009 H1N1 influenza pandemic: insights from modeling, *PLoS Med*, 7, 6.

Weber, M. (1986 [1921]) *The City*. Glencoe: Free Press.

Wenzel, R. (2010) What we learned from H1N1's first year, *The New York Times*, 13 April.

World Health Organization (WHO) (2008) *Cities and Public Health Crises*. Lyons: WHO, available at http://www.who.int/ihr/lyon/FRWHO_HSE_IHR_LYON_2009.5.pdf (accessed 21 April 2012).

9

The making of public health emergencies: West Nile virus in New York City
Sabrina McCormick and Kristoffer Whitney

Introduction

In this chapter we use the case of the West Nile virus (WNV) to investigate the construction of disease-related crises and subsequent changes in public health governance. A mosquito-borne disease first found in Uganda in 1938, which has since been endemic to Africa, the Middle East, India and Indonesia, the WNV was first identified in the United States in New York City during the summer and autumn of 1999 (Asnis *et al.* 2000). While the illness can be severe, it is relatively uncommon and few people who have the antibodies manifest any symptoms. For those who do become symptomatic, manifestations typically include flu-like symptoms, neurological disorders and difficulty breathing. In 1999 New York State experienced 62 cases of encephalitis, meningitis or fever, resulting in seven fatalities.[1] Despite the relative rarity of severe cases, the WNV has become the cause of public health emergency (PHE) declarations in localities across the United States. Millions of US dollars have been spent creating institutional means to fight the disease. While the incidence of the WNV has declined in recent years, international concern about emergent diseases has continued to grow. The WNV was the first disease-based PHE declared in the US at the federal level, and offers a case with which to understand the social construction of PHE.

Our examination of the social construction of crisis emerges from a larger literature on the social construction of illness, which implicates contemporary moral, ethical and political beliefs, the socialisation of medical practitioners, medical institutions and larger social structures in the naming and framing of illness and illness experience (Brown 1995). Illnesses are as much social as biological phenomena. Applying this insight to PHEs implies that a crisis event is not self-evident but a socio-political accomplishment. In the case of the WNV, a crisis was constructed not simply by contemporary medical institutions but also by a suite of pre-existing practices and legal structures involving human, animal and environmental health and risk. Once designated a PHE, the disease altered these structures in ways that allowed the WNV to spread simultaneously as a crisis and as a symbol of similar, future threats. An emergent disease crisis, almost by definition, involves the short term, the unexpected and the uncertain. Because of this, the social construction of a PHE often leads to the circumvention of 'normal' governance regimes, which can potentially marginalise the very populations considered at risk. It is not our purpose to critique New York City's

Pandemics and Emerging Infectious Diseases: The Sociological Agenda, First Edition. Edited by Robert Dingwall, Lily M. Hoffman and Karen Staniland. Chapters © 2013 The Authors. Book Compilation © 2013 Foundation for the Sociology of Health & Illness / John Wiley & Sons Ltd.

response to the emergence of the WNV as a means to decide the 'right' or 'wrong' way to handle crisis, nor are we ascribing any personal motivations to the City's emergency decision-makers. Rather, we are describing the structural biases inherent in the US PHE system and the ways in which crisis, as a social construction, has ramifications for both democratic processes and the public health infrastructure.

Based on the case of the WNV in New York City, we conceptualise two mechanisms involved in the social construction and dissemination of PHEs: (i) crisis interventions that have the potential to marginalise citizens' interaction with the state and (ii) the institutional rearrangement of state agencies stemming from the original crisis issue, resulting in altered networks and practices and drawing heavily upon the crisis as a symbol of similar, future public health threats. The declaration of a PHE in the United States allows public health institutions to recoup their expenses for emergency measures and prepare for ongoing and future disease outbreaks. Such funding also, in combination with pre-existing infrastructures, tends to reinforce the original crisis intervention, 'overdetermining' the continuation of some emergency measures over public opposition.

Sociological studies of epidemics, as well as the abundant literature on governmental responses to disaster and risk, have shed light on the power relations involved in public health governance. Well-known work in the sociological literature on disaster has explored the way in which institutional factors affect the incubation of disasters (Vaughan 1996) and system complexity (Perrow 1984) involved in the generation of these events. Though disaster researchers have examined numerous natural and technological events, far less work has investigated the processes involved in generating disease-based public health crises, relating these events to larger issues of governance (Baehr 2005, Quah 2007, Sanford and Ali 2005, Salehi and Ali 2006). On the other hand, much of the classic and contemporary work on risk, democracy and expertise focuses on public health preparedness and deliberation, with less attention given to moments of disaster, emergency or crisis (Douglas and Wildavsky 1982, Jasanoff 1995, Wraith and Stephenson 2009). We draw upon these complementary perspectives to show that PHE planning is simultaneously a response to moments of crisis construction and a deliberative preparation for future events.

Our first conceptual mechanism, crisis interventions, draws upon the notion of 'states of exception' articulated by Agamben (2005). This describes a state's power to dispense with the normal, legally circumscribed, extent of its authority in times of emergency. An ambiguous state power suggested by constitutional law, allowing for the suspension of that law, a state of exception is a quasi-legal space created in response to crisis with possible consequences for civil liberties. Agamben's work, growing out of a study on the constitutionally granted powers of the state during times of war, has rarely been applied to health emergencies – and when it has been, then only in the context of refugee camps (Nguyen 2009). We argue, however, that there is a family resemblance between Agamben's state of exception and a Federal Emergency Management Agency (FEMA)-type 'state of emergency'. In the story of the WNV's emergence, New York City officials were able to declare a crisis and intervene in ways that were considered heavy-handed and illegal by their critics. This is not to make normative suggestions about whether states should or should not have the power to act in extra-legal ways during extraordinary events, but to draw explicit attention to the ways in which crises are constructed, emergencies are declared and states of exception invoked in the context of disease and public health.

Our second mechanism, institutional rearrangement, draws attention to the processes through which the policies and procedures put in place during emergency declarations ramify, and permanently change the face of public health governance. This process is similar to the ways in which disaster can alter public policy in the wake of what Birkland calls 'focusing events' (1997). Following the construction of the WNV crisis and emergency intervention by New York City, certain techniques of combating the spread of the disease were privileged over others and institutionalised prior to establishing evidence of their efficacy. Furthermore, the power of the WNV as a symbol of future, similar threats helped to instigate changes in a diverse array of federal agencies ostensibly unrelated to managing epidemics. In describing this mechanism, we bring epidemics into discussion with other bodies of literature on the social implications of governmental responses to disaster, terrorism and public participation more generally (Glass and Schoch-Spana 2002, Gottweis 2008).

Methods

This research takes a multi-method approach involving a number of qualitative data collection techniques. We conducted a comprehensive review of the historical scientific construction of the WNV using multiple databases including Medline, Google Scholar and EBSCO, capturing peer-reviewed journals and medical newsletters using search terms related to the WNV. Similarly, we searched the US Federal Register and the Congressional Record from 1999 to the present to capture all government hearings and agency programmes related to the WNV. We also collected media reports using Lexis/Nexis, including newspaper coverage of the WNV from 1999 to the present in the *New York Times* and *The Washington Post*. The Lexis/Nexis legal databases were also utilised to capture court case summaries involving the WNV and mosquito control programmes.

Document collection was followed by semi-structured interviews with three main groups: government officials like first responders and public health officials; medical experts, such as medical examiners and veterinarians; and community members in areas affected by the first WNV outbreaks. An interview schedule was created for each type of interviewee, including issues relevant to each group, such as the diagnostic processes, participation in response programmes and perceptions of illness risk. Initial interviewees were selected based on the literature review and followed by a snowball sampling methodology to capture social actors who fell outside official and expert reports for a total of 22 interviews. The interviews were recorded, transcribed, de-identified and analysed. All uncited quotations are drawn from the anonymous interviews. When dealing with memories of past events and media sources, some inaccuracies and discrepancies are to be expected. However, the details of the events described below were corroborated across data sources (such as interviews and government documents).

Crisis interventions

As indicated above, we conceptualise the response to the WNV as a moment of crisis intervention, followed by institutional rearrangements in the wake of the PHE. To show these temporal dynamics, we divide this largely chronological story at the year 2000, between the initial steps taken to control the WNV by New York City in the first year of its emergence and the institutionalisation of those controls state-wide in the years following.

Initial reaction: New York City, 1999–2000

On 23 August 1999, a doctor at Flushing Hospital in Queens, New York contacted the City Health Department about a small cluster of patients with flu-like symptoms and neurological problems.[2] Initially unable to identify the disease or its sources, the New York City Department of Health and Mental Hygiene (NYCDOH) officials notified the Centers for Disease Control (CDC) in Atlanta, Georgia several days later on 29 August (Senate

Governmental Affairs Committee 2000: 7–8). Initially, five cases – all in Queens – were identified. NYCDOH officials conducted an extensive investigation by first interviewing family members of the patients. Officials found that:

> The only thing we could find in common was that they [the patients] all seemed to like to spend time at home, outdoors, in their gardens, taking little walks, one smoked on the deck, another one stood outside and watched his neighbors' pool get built.

They looked for mosquito breeding grounds in case the illness might be vector-borne. The NYCDOH waited to hear from the CDC for a positive identification of the disease, with St Louis encephalitis, carried from host to host by mosquitoes, being the most likely candidate. Coincidentally, NYCDOH officials and the Office of Emergency Management had been working together on a mass public emergency preparedness test prior to disease emergence, and began to make preparations to engage this system to combat St Louis encephalitis. On 3 September the CDC reported to the City that this disease was indeed the most likely culprit, and in consultation with public health experts New York officials made the decision to launch a full-blown crisis response – including the 'large-scale aerial and ground application of pesticides' for adult mosquitoes (Senate Governmental Affairs committee 2000: 9–12). Within 24 hours a hotline, pesticides, pesticide-spraying airplanes and pilots, cans of N,N-Diethyl-meta-toluamide (DEET), fact sheets, press releases and flyers were mobilised, all coordinated from the emergency command centre at the New York World Trade Center buildings (Covello *et al.* 2001).

While the response was initially limited to airborne and ground spraying of pesticides in northern Queens and the southern Bronx, Mayor Giuliani had mandated the application of the pesticide malathion to 100 per cent of the City by the end of September to control what were still thought to be St. Louis Encephalitis-carrying mosquitoes (Craven and Roehrig 2001, Revkin 1999). This included the outer boroughs being treated twice by air, Manhattan twice by truck, and parts of Queens and the Bronx four times (Fine 2004, Government Accounting Office [GAO] 2000). The City's crisis response also distributed 300,000 cans of DEET and engaged in public education regarding 'risky' activities like being outdoors at dusk, identifying and destroying potential breeding grounds and targeting areas for future spraying (Asnis *et al.* 1999). Simultaneous with the response to human illness was an investigation of seemingly unrelated bird deaths. A local veterinarian sent samples from the dead birds to the US Army's Armed Forces Institute of Pathology for testing. This lab identified the sample as a flavivirus, which led eventually to the correct identification of both the WNV and the connection between the human and animal hosts. By 24 September a 'West Nile-like virus' was identified from the bird specimens and on the 27 September CDC officially reclassified the outbreak as 'West Nile like' – by which time the peak in human cases and the majority of the initial crisis response actions had already taken place (Senate Governmental Affairs committee 2000: 14–17). A comprehensive surveillance system of humans, birds and mosquitoes was instituted to establish infection rates and catch the WNV if it emerged again the following summer.

While human and animal surveillance played an ongoing role in the WNV response, the pesticide spraying campaign produced the most immediate public reaction. Mosquito control had a long history in New York City, beginning with efforts to control malaria in 1901, and including aerial pesticide applications as early as 1956. By the mid-1980s, however, the use of pesticides to control adult mosquitoes had all but ceased (Miller 2001: 359–61). The City's response to WNV/St Louis encephalitis was not unprecedented, therefore, but it was nevertheless a drastic increase in the scale and scope of pesticide use within the living memory of its residents. In anticipation of a public response, the City held news conferences in order to explain the actions it was taking in early September:

> 'We would ask people to understand why we are doing this and to cooperate with us,' [NYC Mayor] Giuliani said . . . as a group of bewildered residents looked on. 'We will do everything we can to try to wipe out the mosquito population and deal with and treat the people who may be bitten and may be affected by it'. (Goodnough 1999)

As the most visible and dramatic response to the disease outbreak, efforts to 'wipe out the mosquito population' with pesticides were heavily emphasised in media reports. Before the precise nature of the disease was known, aerial spraying of pesticides for adult mosquitoes became the public face of the City's disease-control efforts.

While, in retrospect, it was clear that the initial outbreak of the WNV was largely over by October 1999, public debate over New York City's crisis response was just beginning, as the initial confusion over disease identification and the extent of malathion use became known. Local community groups took legal action against New York to oppose the spraying campaigns, claiming that the City's response to the WNV outbreak violated a number of city, state, and federal environmental laws governing water quality. The 'No Spray Coalition', for example, brought a suit against the City by early 2000, charging that the City's 'indiscriminate' spraying was itself a danger to public health and ineffective (US District Court Southern District Court of New York 2007). Such legal contestation reflected how, for many constituencies, the pesticide-spraying programme constituted a greater risk than the disease itself. The technological infrastructure for spraying, however, had been re-established within the first month of the mosquito-borne crisis.

Response institutionalisation: New York State 2000–2001
On 11 October 2000 FEMA declared a State of Emergency for New York.[3] This declaration provided reimbursement for the spraying campaigns carried out in the fall of 1999 and the summer of 2000, and resulted in the approval of funds for other counties in the state as the virus spread. Local departments were able to draw 75 per cent of funding for any WNV-related activities from federal funds up to a total of $5 million. From 1999 to 2000 the NYCDOH spending for surveillance and viral control increased from $1.5 to $7.5 million (Fine 2004). Formal declarations of emergency and disaster are well-worn avenues for seeking financial aid for public health interventions. As one New York City official noted:

> It's city funding, and then eventually you declare your disaster, and then you know the state has to declare a disaster, and then the federal government will reimburse you.

The declaration of a PHE also, however, reinforces the initial state response to crisis; a dynamic that became apparent as the City and State of New York began to formalise their response into an institutionalised programme. In early 2000 the City and the State of New York began to draft and solicit public comment on the State DOH's 'West Nile virus response plan' and the NYCDOH's 'Adult mosquito control programs draft environmental impact statement'. As with the initial public outcry over mosquito spraying in late 1999, activist opposition to these formal plans centred around a few prominent issues. Critics questioned the necessity and efficacy of the initial spray campaign, complained of poor public notification procedures for the spraying, expressed scepticism about the safety of the chosen insecticides and their application, questioned the City's claim that the risk of contracting the WNV outweighed that of pesticide exposure and insisted that the models that the City was using to predict pesticide spray drift were inadequate (New York City Department of Health 2000, 2001, New York State Department of Health [NYSDOH] 2000a, 2000b). As one interviewee based in Long Island summarised these concerns:

> They're doing this in an effort to control a population of mosquitoes that science tells us you can't control, and they're doing it as a disease management prevention strategy, when nobody's dying.

The uncertainty surrounding pesticide use was repeatedly stressed by opponents. As one environmental advocate commented in response to the City's 'Draft environmental impact statement':

> Given the sparseness of information available to estimate risk from pesticides . . . and the lack of a true control scenario with which to make disease estimates . . . the process is simply not capable of making a definitive judgment one way or the other on this question. (NYCDOH 2001: 45)

To these organisations, precaution in the face of uncertainty lay in refusing to spray. For many public health officials, however, a precautionary approach suggested aggressive pesticide spraying to avoid a large-scale outbreak of the WNV. As a governmental report to the US Congress put it:

> Because New York City had ceased active mosquito surveillance and control in the late 1980s . . . the city had no way to determine where mosquitoes were living and breeding. Faced with the need to reduce mosquito populations very quickly, the city immediately began large-scale aerial and ground application of pesticides. (Senate Governmental Affairs committee 2000: 12)

In the case of the WNV, as other scholars have also pointed out, 'precaution points two ways' (Scott 2005, Tickner 2002). Note that these concerns were not solely raised in the deliberative risk management process that a response 'plan' would suggest, but also as a post hoc debate on crisis interventions that had already taken place. As New York City, the State and the CDC all assessed their response to the WNV and sought public comment in 2000 and 2001, the debate looked both backwards and forward in time – seeking to justify or undermine the initial crisis response and shape future emergency planning.

These plans, as eventually adopted, would seem to have found a precautionary middle ground, making adult mosquito spraying a last resort in a hierarchical approach that stressed education, surveillance and larvicides ahead of using aerial pesticides. As the Long Island organisation Citizens' Campaign for the Environment pointed out, however, the practical realities of New York's PHE system stood this hierarchy on its head. The Campaign took issue with the state's insistence that it was advocating spraying only as a 'last resort', by arguing that because most funding was tied to the declaration of a 'public health threat' local action was in reality biased toward spraying and away from more benign preventative measures:

> Currently, DOH pays the highest amount for adult mosquito spraying and the least for education and larval control. Under this current approach, state funding provides a financial incentive for high impact chemical use and nothing for benign activities or education. (Westchester County Government 2002)

When this issue was raised in public comment on the State's WNV response plan, officials were forced to admit that their hands were tied by public health legislation:

> Reimbursement rates for mosquito and vector control and public health threats are specified in Public Health Law (Sections 611, 605) or regulations (10 NYCRR Part 44) and the Plan must be structured within these parameters. (NYSDOH 2001: 60)

While New York prescribed a plan in the wake of the WNV controversy that placed priority on education and surveillance, the deeper structure of PHEs preferentially funded the initial response: pesticide spraying. Historical, technological and legal infrastructures combined to reinforce the construction of the WNV crisis as a PHE and institutionalised the controversial spraying of adulticides.

Institutional rearrangement

In the years following the initial 1999 outbreak, the WNV spread across the United States. The situation that obtained in New York played out similarly in many locales across the country. The disease not only instituted changes in public health administration but served as a source of funding and motivation to make changes in a number of governmental agencies, some ostensibly unrelated to managing epidemics. As a PHE, the WNV could serve as a symbol of future outbreaks and similar threats. And through the symbolic leveraging of the WNV, agencies as diverse as the CDC, the US Fish and Wildlife Service (FWS), the US Geological Survey (USGS), and the National Aeronautics and Space Administration (NASA) have utilised this PHE to garner funds, establish new interagency networks and create new programmes of research, intervention and surveillance. This was done neither lightly nor surreptitiously, but in response to what government officials considered the wake-up call of the WNV crisis. Early federal government assessment reports were explicit on this score, noting the convergence of human and animal health investigators on the identification of the disease, calling for increased cooperation between human and animal disease laboratories and surveillance systems, and associating the WNV with epidemic disease and the threat of bioterrorism more generally (Senate Governmental Affairs Committee 2000, GAO 2000).

The US *Federal Register*, as the official journal of the federal government and clearinghouse for public information, is a window onto the widespread concern over the WNV in the wake of the original crisis. During the first few years after the outbreak in New York, roughly 1999–2002, the WNV received attention from a relatively limited number of federal agencies concerned with emergent disease, human and animal surveillance programmes, potential vaccine development and the screening of blood donations. As attention to non-human hosts and mosquito vectors had proven integral to the identification and surveillance of the WNV in New York City, agencies like the CDC offered funding for research explicitly focused on the movement of birds, virus transmission, and improved disease prevention (for example, Department of Health and Human Services 2001). The Government Accounting Office (2000) analysis of governmental response to the WNV, in fact, had claimed that a lack of coordination between the human-centred and animal-centred agencies slowed responses. As a result, physicians and public health officials explicitly worked to better integrate communication between animal and human health agencies – a first wave of institutional rearrangement.

After 2003, the appearance of the WNV in the *Federal Register* reflected a new emphasis by a greater diversity of agencies. The WNV went from an object of direct study (for example, funding from the CDC for WNV vaccine research) to an example of a type of risk (for example, emergent diseases and bioterrorism). In addition, the WNV ramified beyond animal to human transmission concerns to include risk solely to animals. For example, the FWS began to routinely list the WNV as a possible threat to species being considered for threatened or endangered status. After 2004 the WNV frequently appeared in such FWS announcements, as well as in US Food and Drug Administration meeting agendas addressing the potential infectious disease risks to the nation's blood supply. From 2005 on, in fact, these two agencies make up the bulk of WNV appearances in the *Federal Register*. Since 1999 the WNV has become an object of research, a potential source of funding, and a symbol of concern across multiple public health and animal health institutions in the US government, well beyond its original geographical and institutional scope.

After 2003 governmental officials also began to stress similar illnesses that might emerge in the future. The WNV response was increasingly conceptualised as a model for disease outbreaks of other kinds, and the surveillance systems put in place to detect the WNV were also argued to be critical for the detection of other emergent illnesses. These new networks and programmes were based upon both the spread of the disease and the symbolic power of a potential epidemic. This power helped to create what officials have called the most comprehensive vector-borne disease surveillance system in US history. The ArboNET/ Plague Surveillance System is a collaboration between CDC, the USGS, NASA and nationwide local health departments that map diseases in real-time in order to make predictions of a disease outbreak. The system's origins are in a plague surveillance system developed in 1981, but funding and support increased exponentially following the emergence of the WNV. The rationale for this system, according to one federal public health official, was that the WNV outbreak:

> was a unique situation in the sense that it was the first large-scale incursion of a vector borne disease in recent years into North America. And because these are primarily zoonotic diseases, or primarily, in this case a disease of birds, it really did require a coordinated response like never before.

While the WNV provided an important catalyst, programmes like the ArboNET/Plague Surveillance System are directed at a larger range of illnesses including Ebola Hemorrhagic fever and Rift Valley fever. As one of the lead administrators at NASA stated publicly:

> NASA satellite remote sensing technology has been an important tool in the last few years to not only provide scientists with the data needed to respond to epidemic threats quickly, but to also help predict the future of infectious diseases in areas where diseases were never a main concern. (*American Society of Tropical Medicine and Hygiene* 2007)

The WNV, as both crisis and symbol of emergent disease, has prompted a wide variety of state interventions, responses and rearrangements, with ramifications so far removed from its emergence in New York City as to belie any explicit relationship between, say, NASA satellites and the death of crows in Queens.

Conclusion

Our aim in this chapter has not been to adjudicate the correct response to the WNV but to explore how the social construction of crisis and other moments of disease-related PHE function on an institutional level. While we have utilised public criticism of New York City's pesticide spraying campaign to analyse the relationship between crisis interventions and public participation in emergency response, it is important to point out that resistance to such measures is not universal. Groups at risk for an emergent illness may well want their government officials to act quickly and decisively against potential epidemics. However, the construction of crisis as a state of emergency – a notion from legal theory that we have transposed from Agamben's 'state of exception' – allows those in power to assert social and technological control over populations by implementing practices that would, under normal circumstances, require public deliberation. Indeed, PHEs explicitly and structurally link funding for public health governance with the ability to enact potentially marginalising crisis interventions. These interventions not only proceed with little or no public input, but outlast the initial moment of crisis to become the structurally favoured solution thereafter.

We acknowledge the limited nature of the choices available to the New York DOH. The WNV 'state of exception' ostensibly gave the City broad discretionary powers; yet, in reality, the options were limited by prior institutional structures – in this case, aerial spraying for adult mosquitoes was an important historical method for controlling these disease vectors. Almost by definition, emergency measures are undertaken without considering structural biases, alternatives, legal review or public opinion; a point made repeatedly by critics of New York City's spraying policies. It is also important to note, however, that alternatives did exist; a fact that became increasingly evident as the WNV spread outward from New York and other municipalities had to make choices about how to intervene. To briefly take one example, in 2000 the state of Connecticut conducted a far more limited spraying campaign despite recording thousands of bird deaths, and felt justified in their restraint by a very low rate of human infection. As a state epidemiologist stated publicly: 'We only sprayed on three occasions. As it turns out, we probably did the right thing' (Ruane 2001). Although there were constraints on the choice of reactions to the WNV, blanket aerial spraying of mosquito adulticides was not the only option available to local departments of health.

Risk scholar Sheila Jasanoff (1996) has made the political separation of experts and citizens one of the key, unresolved tensions of the modern state:

> To serve as a basis for collective action, scientific knowledge has to be produced in tandem with social legitimation. Insulating the experts in closed worlds of formal inquiry and then, under the label of participation, opening up their findings to unlimited critical scrutiny appears to be a recipe for unending debate and spiraling distrust. This is the core dilemma of environmental democracy. (Jasanoff 1996: 69)

WNV court cases surrounding the City's pesticide applications point up this dilemma quite clearly. Lobster fishers who brought suit against the manufacturers of the pesticides involved, for example, had a very different perspective on the decision to spray than did the defendants. To the fishers, 'City officials, although not at that stage believing that the situation presented a true emergency, decided to spray the entire city of New York twice with pesticides' (Fox v Cheminova, Inc. 2005). The chemical company, on the other hand, believed that 'on September 3, 1999, trained experts made an informed decision to administer the pesticides given the state of emergency' (Fox v Cheminova, Inc. 2005). The 'emergency' was not a given but rather a complicated social construction made up of uncertain disease and vector characteristics, financial, technological and epistemological commitments, and sociopolitical status. Understanding the bureaucratic context within which PHEs are constructed, altered and reproduced is a key component for promoting democratic deliberation on how crises should be addressed and what emergency powers the state should have the right to exercise. It is not impugning any one individual or collective motivation to suggest, as scholars have been doing for years, that lay involvement in public health debate is both good politics and good science (Brown 1993), or that technocratic decisionism can preempt citizens' rights to make ethical and technical choices (Wynne 1997). As public hearings are simultaneously planning for the future and adjudicating the past, so scholarly critique of historical events like the WNV crisis can aid in public deliberation over the definition and enactment of future PHEs. As emergent disease continues to be an important health concern worldwide, it is our hope that the WNV case can serve as a basis for ongoing, explicit discussion of the construction of crisis.

Acknowledgements

The authors would like to acknowledge the Robert Wood Johnson Foundation for supporting this research, and thank Robert Aronowitz and the reviewers and editors at SHI for their thoughtful comments on earlier versions of this chapter.

Notes

1   These are the retrospective official numbers from the Department of Health and Human Services, Centers for Disease Control and Prevention (2001).
2   Queens is the most easterly of five boroughs of New York City that contains an ethnically and economically diverse population.
3   This declaration, together with a similar declaration for New Jersey a month later, represent the only Federal-level emergency declarations for 'virus threat'. See the searchable Federal Emergency Management Agency (n.d.).

References

Agamben, G. (2005) *State of Exception*. Chicago: University of Chicago Press.
American Society of Tropical Medicine and Hygiene (2007) NASA technology helps predict and prevent future pandemic outbreaks, *ScienceDaily*, Available at http://www.science daily.com/releases/2007/11/071106140029.htm (accessed 15 November 2012).
Asnis, D., Conetta, R., Waldman, G. and Teixeira, A. *et al.* (1999) Outbreak of West Nile-like viral encephalitis: New York, 1999, *Morbidity and Mortality Weekly Report*, 48, 38, 845–9.
Asnis, D., Conetta, R., Teixeira, A. and Waldman, G. *et al.* (2000) The West Nile virus outbreak of 1999 in New York: the Flushing Hospital Experience, *Clinical Infectious Diseases*, 30, 5, 413–18.
Baehr, P. (2005) Social extremity, communities of fate, and the sociology of SARS, *European Journal of Sociology*, 46, 2, 179–211.
Birkland, T.A. (1997) *After Disaster: Agenda Setting, Public Policy, and Focusing Events*. Washington, DC: Georgetown University Press.
Brown, P. (1993) When the public knows better: popular epidemiology challenges the system, *Environment*, 35, 8, 16–41.
Brown, P. (1995) Naming and framing: the social construction of diagnosis and illness, *Journal of Health and Social Behavior*, 36, Special issue, 34–52.
Covello, V.T., Peters, R.G., Wojtecki, J.G. and Hyde, R.C. (2001) Risk communication: the West Nile virus epidemic, and bioterrorism: responding to the communication challenges posed by the inten-

tional or unintentional release of a pathogen in an urban setting, *Journal of Urban Health*, 78, 2, 382–91.

Craven, R.B. and Roehrig, J.T. (2001) West Nile virus, *Journal of the American Medical Association*, 286, 6, 651–3.

Department of Health and Human Services, Centers for Disease Control and Prevention (2001) Applied Research in Emerging Infections Investigations of West Nile Virus; Notice of Availability of Funds, *Federal Register*, 66, 100: 28522–3.

Douglas, M. and Wildavsky, A. (1982) *Risk and Culture: An Essay on the Selection of Technical and Environmental Dangers*. Berkeley, CA: University of California Press.

Federal Emergency Management Agency (n.d.) Database at: http://www.fema.gov/news/disasters. fema (accessed 27 May 2011).

Fine, A. (2004) *Sustaining Surveillance for West Nile Virus in New York City, 1999–(2004)*. New York: New York City Department of Health and Mental Hygiene.

Fox v Cheminova, Inc. (2005) 00-CV-5145 (TCP)(ETB), United States District Court for the Eastern District of New York, 387 F. Supp. 2d 160; (2005) US Dist. LEXIS 19915, August 25, (2005) Decided, Motion granted by, in part, Motion denied by, in part Fox v. Cheminova, Inc., (2006) US Dist. LEXIS 11463 (E.D.N.Y., Mar. 1, (2006)).

Gottweis, H. (2008) Participation and the new governance of life. *Biosocieties*, 3, 3, 265–86.

Government Accounting Office (GAO) (2000) *West Nile Virus Outbreak: Lessons for Public Health Preparedness*. Washington: US Government Printing Office.

Glass, T. and Schoch-Spana, M. (2002) Bioterrorism and the people: how to vaccinate a city against panic, *Clinical Infectious Diseases*, 34, 2, 217–23.

Goodnough, A. (1999) Encephalitis strikes 3 people, 1 fatally, in Queens, City says. New York Times, A1. September 4. Available at http://www.nytimes.com/1999/09/04/nyregion/encephalitis-strikes-3-people-1-fatally-in-queens-city-says.html (accessed 15 November 2012).

Jasanoff, S. (1996) The dilemma of environmental democracy, *Issues in Science and Technology*, 63–70.

Jasanoff, S. (1995) *Science at the Bar: Law, Science, and Technology in America*. Cambridge: Harvard University Press.

Miller, J.R. (2001) The control of mosquito-borne diseases in New York City, *Journal of Urban Health*, 78, 2, 359–66.

New York City Department of Health (NYCDOH) (2000) Appendix A: Response to Comments on the Draft Scope of Analysis. Adult mosquito control programs draft environmental impact statement: New York. Available at http://home2.nyc.gov/html/doh/downloads/pdf/wnv/comments.pdf (accessed 15 November 2012).

NYCDOH (2001) *Chapter 6: Response to comments on the DEIS*. Adult mosquito control programs final environmental impact statement. New York. Available at http://www.nyc.gov/html/doh/html/wnv/feis.shtml (accessed 15 November 2102).

New York State Department of Health (NYSDOH) (2000a) Draft New York State West Nile Virus response plan, February 18. New York.

NYSDOH (2000b) New York State West Nile virus response plan, May. New York.

NYSDOH (2001) New York State West Nile Virus response plan – guidance document, May. New York.

Nguyen, V.K. (2009) Government-by-exception: enrolment and experimentality in mass HIV treatment programmes in Africa, *Social Theory & Health*, 7, 196–217.

Perrow, C. (1984) *Normal Accidents: Living with High Risk Technologies*. New York: Basic Books.

Quah, S.R. (2007) Public image and governance of epidemics: comparing HIV/AIDS and SARS, *Health Policy* 80, 2, 253–72.

Revkin, A. (1999) As mosquito spraying continues, officials stress its safety. *New York Times*. Available at http://www.nytimes.com/1999/09/14/nyregion/as-mosquito-spraying-continues-officials-stress-its-safety.html?pagewanted=all&src=pm (accessed 18 January 2012).

Ruane, M.E. (2001) Watching and waiting for the West Nile virus. 15 April. C01. The Washington Post.

Salehi, R. and Ali, S. (2006) The social and political context of disease outbreaks: the case of SARS in Toronto, *Canadian Public Policy/Analyse de Politiques*, 32, 4, 373–85.

Sanford, S. and Ali, H. (2005) The new public health hegemony: response to acute respiratory syndrome (SARS) in Toronto, *Social Theory & Health*, 3, 105–25.

Scott, D. (2005) When precaution points two ways: confronting 'West Nile fever', *Canadian Journal of Law and Society*, 20, 2, 27–65.

Senate Governmental Affairs Committee (2000) Expect the unexpected: the West Nile virus wake up call. Report of the Minority Staff to Senator Joseph Lieberman, Ranking Member. Available at http://www.ntis.gov/search/product.aspx?ABBR=PB2001101067 (accessed 15 November 2012).

Tickner, J.A. (2002) The precautionary principle and public health trade-offs: case study of West Nile virus, *Annals of the American Academy of Political and Social Science*, 584, 1, 69–79.

US Centers for Disease Control and Prevention (2001) Adult Mosquitos Control Program Final Impact Statement. Available at: http://www.cdc.gov/ncidod/dvbid/westnile/surv&controlCase Count99_detailed.htm (Accessed 29 February 2012).

US District Court, Southern District of New York (2007) No Spray Coalition, Inc. v the City of New York, Stipulation of Agreement and Order. 00 Civ. 5395 (GBD) (RLE) New York.

Vaughan, D. (1996) *The Challenger Launch Decision: Risky Technology, Culture, and Deviance at NASA*. Chicago: University of Chicago Press.

Westchester County Government (2002) Chapter 4: response to comments on the DGEIS. Available at http://www.westchestergov.com/hdbooklets/StingEIS/FGEISfiles/Chapter4.pdf (accessed 21 November 2012).

Wraith, C. and Stephenson, N. (2009) Risk, insurance, preparedness and the disappearance of the population: the case of pandemic influenza, *Health Sociology Review*, 18, 4, 220–33.

Wynne, B. (1997) Methodology and Institutions: value as seen from the risk field. In Foster, J. (ed.) *Valuing Nature?: Ethics, Economics and the Environment*. New York: Routledge.

10

Using model-based evidence in the governance of pandemics

Erika Mansnerus

One need no longer have recourse to magic means to master or implore the spirits, as did the savage, for whom the mysterious powers existed. Technical means and calculations perform the service. (Max Weber in Gerth and Wright Mills 1958: 117)

Introduction

The worst nightmares of public health officials could have been realised by a pandemic outbreak in 2009. A globally widespread new mutation of the 'swine flu' A/H1N1 influenza virus put pre-pandemic plans to the test, urging citizens to respond to the threat through heightened hygiene levels and voluntary quarantine or travel restrictions. These mitigation strategies were supported by model-based estimates of transmission rates for the outbreak.

The life-threatening nature of a pandemic triggers various responses. Previous studies have analysed media representations of pandemics, the metaphors associated with the communication of pandemics and the legitimation of pandemic preparedness planning (Garoon and Duggan 2008, Nerlich and Halliday 2007, Stephenson and Jamieson 2009, Wallis and Nerlich 2005). However, the pandemic narrative itself, as Leach and Dry suggest, can be told by different voices in order to raise questions of power and social justice (Leach and Dry 2010, see also Stirling and Scoones 2009). Narrative is not just a story, but a story with a specific purpose and consequences.

The idea of models as narratives, or modelling as a mode of storytelling, is acknowledged as a useful metaphor in understanding the mathematical machinery (Gramelsberger 2010, Morgan 2001). Models tell a story that can explain a phenomenon, predict the course of an outbreak or provide an assessment of the efficacy of preventive measures. Stories have a purpose and are told to a particular audience. They are a way to understand how modelling functions in pandemic governance.

This chapter examines the evidence produced by pre-pandemic and pandemic modelling as narratives and analyses how those narratives gain quantitative authority despite the uncertainties embodied in mathematical modelling. The pre-pandemic narrative describes how an outbreak might occur and proposes mitigation strategies. A pandemic narrative shows how well computational techniques respond to the outbreak situation and accommodate uncertainties. Does modelling become a magic means, in Weber's phrase?

Quantitative authority, according to Espeland and Stevens (2008), is built on the persuasiveness of numerical information. Quantitative authority, or the authority of numbers, derives from four attitudes adopted from Desrosières (1998 in Espeland and Stevens 2008: 419): the sense of numbers as accurate or valid representations of the world; their usefulness in solving problems; their capacity to link users who have investments in numbers, and their association with rationality and objectivity. Along with these four attitudes, Espeland and Stevens (2008: 421) note that the:

> authority of numbers can be investigated through their practical uses; describing how they become embedded in networks of people who make and use them, and the techniques and routines that facilitate this embedding.

This applies Latour's approach as to the construction of scientific facts to governance by numbers (for example, Latour and Woolgar 1986, Pinch and Bijker 1984). In this sense, quantitative authority acknowledges the mutual construction of statistical knowledge and social order (for example, Jasanoff 2004, Rudinow Saetnan et al. 2011). It establishes 'reliance on quantifiable objects', in Porter's (2000: 226) phrase.

Computations translate uncertainties into the tangible, the numerical and the quantifiable (Desrosières 1998, Power 1997, Strathern 2000). When models gain quantitative authority, they become 'forms and tools of calculation' (Dean 2010: 42) in the sense of technical rationality, *techne*. I understand *techne* as the processes and practices of calculation that transform and produce knowledge in order to make sense of it, to organise and govern, perhaps even to anticipate risks and uncertainties by numerical means. The notion itself is the third axis of governmentality, as Dean (2010) interprets Foucault's work.

Methods of analysis
This study discusses a set of pre-pandemic models (Bootsma and Ferguson 2007, Ferguson et al. 2006, Hatchett et al. 2007) studied during an introductory course to modelling methods at the London School for Hygiene and Tropical Medicine in June 2007. During the 2009 pandemic I followed risk assessment reports published by the European Disease Control Centre (EDCC). These showed how modelling methods were used to govern the pandemic outbreak. I also studied a set of early pandemic models (Fraser et al. 2009, Garske et al. 2009, Lipsitch et al. 2009), presented and discussed in a seminar, 'Healthy Futures', at the University of Cambridge in January 2010. Their influence was traced through citation analysis. Finally, I examined the official UK evaluation of policy responses to the 2009 outbreak (Hine 2010). The analysis of these documents was informed by Prior's (2006: 91) view of the productivity of documents, which means treating the document 'as topic rather than as resource' and tracing their effects.

Modelling pandemics: How do models tell their stories?

Prior to the actual declaration of a global pandemic, preparedness planning developed modelling techniques. In these pre-pandemic narratives the 1918 Spanish flu provided a historical point of reference to assess applicable mitigation strategies. These narratives are grounded in past data but give us future predictions. By analysing how the pre-pandemic models tell stories we learn what kind of entities models are and how they gain quantitative authority.

Modelling helps us make inferences that go beyond direct observation. The underlying idea of 'extending beyond bounds of direct observation' not only characterises epidemiological reasoning, as Hampton Frost (1965 in Snow: ix) initially observed, but it also captures the nature of modelling. Models can be seen as scientific instruments (for example, like a microscope) designed for investigation, measurement and experimentation (Morgan 2001, 2012, Fox Keller 2000, 2003). Some studies emphasise their unfolding and multiplex nature and their mediatory roles (Merz 1999, Morgan and Morrison 1999). Models can be seen as a bridge between theory and practice, as Den Butter and Morgan suggest (2000). For them, a model is not only a scientific object but also constitutes expertise and enables normative knowledge to be gained. Models, in this sense, seem to occupy a dual role: they are not solely operating on the scientific domain but also provide evidence to policy processes (for example, Landström et al. 2011, van Egmond and Zeiss 2010, Yearley 1999).

Epidemiological models are typically built to address particular research questions that originate from policy-driven initiatives (for example, Habbema et al. 1996). We can say that they are tailored. Tailoring a model simply means building and using a model for a particular purpose. This metaphor was used in a seminar at the University of Helsinki in October 2001, during a previous study, by a senior scientist who described at length the relationship between a modeller and a customer: model-building was a response to the customer's needs.

Pre-pandemic models are models of large-scale infectious diseases that predict a possible outbreak and test public health interventions in order to contain or restrict the transmission. These interventions can be either pharmaceutical (PI) or non-pharmaceutical (NPI). They typically use available data from past pandemics (1918 and 1957) but also incorporate geographical data for spatial simulations. My analysis of the pre-pandemic models identified three elements that constitute an infectious disease model: data, computational techniques and epidemiological understanding of the infection.

Model parameterisation is dependent on data. In epidemiological modelling, data are derived from surveillance activities or field studies. Surveillance activities are carried out on various levels: on a national level by public health institutes, such as the Health Protection Agency in the UK and the Institute for Health and Welfare in Finland; on an international level by the ECDC in Stockholm, and on an inter-governmental level by the World Health Organization (WHO), especially through the Global Outbreak Alert and Response Network (2009, 2011). When modelling happens during the early days of a pandemic outbreak, data may not be available. In some cases, data may have been collected for different purposes, such as for earlier surveys or statistical analyses. In this case, parameter estimation may not be fully supported by data, which leaves uncertainties in the model. Based on the estimates, the model calculates high and moderate transmissibility scenarios for outbreaks. Mathematical algorithms, which are chosen to reflect the dynamics of the transmission process as closely as possible, direct the execution of the simulations.

The pre-pandemic models studied the efficacy of NPI and PI during a pandemic outbreak. NPI include school closures, travel restrictions, bans on public gatherings and quarantine (or case isolation). The effectiveness of public health interventions during the 1918 influenza pandemic in the US was modelled.

The main story from these models is that significant reduction in influenza transmission can be achieved only by the rapid and simultaneous implementation of several NPIs. School closures should be accompanied by travel restrictions and case isolation or quarantine. The model findings emphasise that the 'aggressive' implementation of [NPIs as mitigation strategies] flattens the curve and reduces the number of infectious cases. Importantly, the models also warn that relaxing the NPIs is likely to increase the spread of the virus (Hatchett *et al.* 2007: 7584).

When is it safe to relax the interventions? In the event of a severe pandemic, NPIs need to be held in place for longer than the 2–8 weeks that was the practice in 1918. This time window is dependent on how quickly emergency vaccines are produced. Implementing the recommendations from this narrative is not, however, straightforward. Long-term school closure, travel restrictions or quarantine all have a socioeconomic impact (for example, Smith *et al.* 2011). Moreover, pandemics are known to manifest as a two-peak curve: after the initial outbreak, a second wave is expected. Uncertainty about the duration of the pandemic makes it difficult to follow the recommendations from the pre-pandemic narratives.

In order to mitigate the severity of a new influenza pandemic the task of pre-pandemic, large-scale simulation models was to map the complex landscape of intervention strategies. A model representing the transmission of influenza in households, schools and workplaces was parameterised on the basis of population density data and data from travel patterns (Ferguson *et al.* 2006). In the parameterisation, the transmission rate was assumed to follow that of the 1918 influenza pandemic. From this modelled narrative, we learn that the isolation of infected cases and household quarantine are effective measures, whereas travel restrictions have only a very small effect in delaying the outbreak. These pre-pandemic stories were listened to in 2009 when the swine flu pandemic hit the headlines. As part of the pandemic guidelines, the WHO issued a statement that travel restrictions were unnecessary, yet individuals followed their own judgement and reduced travel to affected countries in the early days of the outbreak (WHO 2009).

These stories were criticised for their assumptions that there will be no 'spontaneous change in the behaviour of an uninfected individuals as the pandemic progresses' during a pandemic, though 'increased social distance' has been reported, as Ferguson *et al.* (2006: 448) note. A virtual game world allowed a different story to emerge. In September 2005 an outbreak affected an estimated population of 4 million people. This epidemic, unknown to us who are familiar with 1918, 1957 and 1968 pandemics, took place in a virtual world, an online role playing game called World of Warcraft (Blizzard Entertainment, Irvine CA, USA). The outbreak was caused by a disease called Corrupted Blood, which mimicked the transmission patterns of the great pandemics. In their analysis of the anatomy of this virtual outbreak, Lofgren and Fefferman show how virtual outbreaks in games work as a large-scale experiment that overcomes physical, ethical and financial restrictions (Lofgren and Fefferman 2007). The same could be said about any simulation model but virtual game worlds can go a step further than mathematical models. In a virtual world, subjects are virtual but their actions are controlled by human players. This is a crucial difference from pandemic simulation models, which make fairly fixed assumptions of human behaviour. Yet, their advantages may be questioned: how reliable is the virtual behaviour of humans in a game world? Balicer found that the risk-taking behaviour of the virtual characters is dependent on the rules and goals of the game (Balicer 2007). But these virtual playgrounds emphasise an important aspect often missing in simulation models; namely, the need to understand the complexity of human behaviour at the time of an outbreak.

Despite their limitations, these pre-pandemic narratives serve as predictive scenarios, as possible accounts of what might happen. They provide representations of the world that are as accurate as possible, which is one of the attitudes that increases their persuasiveness (Mansnerus 2012). In their quantitative form, pre-pandemic models gained enough authority to encourage a relaxed policy on travel restrictions. However, these narratives give a narrow view on how people behave during an outbreak. This is partly due to a lack of data on behavioural patterns, although there are now attempts to use mobile phone or Internet analytic data to remedy this. It is also partly due to the computational restrictions on modelling that make behavioural data difficult to incorporate, especially when it comes to identifying relevant metrics for the transformation of qualitative observations into the quantitative terms that modelling requires. The key function of pre-pandemic models seems to be their capacity to inform strategic planning and risk assessment.

Accommodating uncertainties in modelled narratives of pandemics

When the 2009 swine flu outbreak was declared a pandemic by WHO, a narrative was urgently needed for policy-making. Modelling was used to clarify how serious the outbreak would be, and how best to design interventions, as soon as any data from the earliest cases in Mexico were available. A group of modellers (Fraser *et al.* 2009) analysed the early data on the virus's international spread and genetic diversity in the WHO Informal Modelling Network. Their collaboration was facilitated by teleconferencing and face-to-face meetings (personal communication January 2010). The findings suggested that the virus would be clinically less severe than the 1918 virus and that transmissibility was higher than that of seasonal flu. Interestingly, the main emphasis of this early assessment was uncertainty, due to the limited or unavailable data needed for the parameterisation of the model:

> To reduce all these uncertainties, it is essential that public health agencies around the world continue to collect high-quality epidemiological data. (Fraser *et al.* 2009: 1561).

Despite the uncertainty, this model gained quantitative authority as a key reference point with 548 citations (ISI Web of Knowledge) compared to the two other models under scrutiny (Lipsitch *et al.* 2009: 61 citations; Garske *et al.* 2009: 57 citations).

The modelling exercise informed the change in UK policy from local containment to the national management of a widespread pandemic. Various mitigation strategies were implemented. The best known were distribution of antiviral medications through an National Health Service helpline; online self-assessment and 'flu buddy' arrangements, where a nominated friend, family member or neighbour was able to fetch antiviral treatment from a pharmacy. The WHO declaration of a pandemic alert Phase 6 prompted a series of governmental actions. Vaccine development began as soon as the virus was isolated and vaccinations were available from September 2009, initially targeting risk groups with a lowered immune response or at a higher risk of encountering the infection. In the UK the vaccine uptake was not high – about 37 per cent of the population, according to the Department of Health (2010) – mainly because the pandemic was fairly mild. In total, it led to fewer than 20,000 deaths worldwide, as documented by the WHO (2011).[1]

In Finland the pandemic happened on a smaller scale. The main difference was that the vaccine uptake was higher (up to 49 per cent of the population, reaching 77 per cent among children), with people queuing for hours to get vaccinated. The aftermath of the pandemic was worse than in the UK. In the winter of 2010 an increased number of narcolepsy cases among children were documented. In 2012 the Finnish health authorities and the European Centre for Disease Prevention and Control documented an association between the Pandemrix vaccine (GlaxoSmithKline, London, UK) and the onset of narcolepsy (Institute for Health and Welfare 2011, ECDC 2012).

Uncertainties, about the unpredictable mutability and virulence of the pathogen, the availability of data and the safety of PIs, shape this storyline. Uncertainty need not necessarily undermine the science: it can also be a source of heterogeneity and richness for the evidence-base offered to policymakers, as Shackley and Wynne (1996) suggest in their study of representations of uncertainty in climate science and policy. More recently, model uncertainties have been reclassified in terms of levels and dimensions, which acknowledge parameter and structural uncertainties as parts of a more complex account of limited knowledge, indeterminacies and ignorance (Spiegelhalter and Riesch 2011, Wynne 1992).

Uncertainties, however, may be embedded in the pandemic narrative as a result of missing or incomplete evidence when the model is being built. These uncertainties are reminiscent of MacKenzie's (1990: 370–371) 'certainty trough', where uncertainty about a technical object (in that case a missile), was lower for the users than for the producers. They are acknowledged as 'known unknowns' in the narratives that assess pandemic risks, for example, the ECDC Pandemic Risk Assessment reports (Prevention 2009a, 2009b). Three unknown factors are:

- those related to the microbiological factors
- those related to the lack of precise parameters for modelling and forecasting purposes
- those related to the effectiveness and safety of PIs

The ECDC report in September 2009 notes that 'pandemic viruses are unpredictable and can change their characteristics as they evolve and, perhaps, reassort with other influenza viruses'. This creates microbiological 'uncertainty' that affects model-based risk assessment, but is also acknowledged in the pre-pandemic narratives, which state the unknown nature of the virulence and mutability of the pathogen. Once the virus is isolated, this uncertainty eases, though the viral response to antiviral pharmaceuticals remains unknown (ECDC 2009a).

One of the key questions for models was the speed with which the outbreak would spread (Fraser et al. 2009). These estimates become another source of uncertainty. An estimate of transmission, which is a quantifiable variable, is calculated as a basic reproductive rate.[2] The rate shows the average number of individuals directly infected by a single infectious case. When estimating the transmission rate for a pandemic, the underlying assumption is that the whole population is susceptible to the infection. For the A/H1N1 viral outbreak, the reproductive rate was estimated to be 1.5–2. By comparison, the reproductive rate for a seasonal influenza is 1.1–1.2, and for measles, it is higher than 10 (Nicoll and Coulombier 2009). These estimates show how many clinical cases, that is, infected individuals, there are in relation to one case in a fully susceptible population.

Estimating the reproductive rate brings uncertainty to the models. It is not certain how virulent the pathogen is in the early days of the pandemic when the virus is not yet isolated, or during pre-pandemic modelling when estimates rely on past data. There may also be uncertainty about the susceptibility of the population. Recent research suggests the co-evolution of human populations and pathogens, such that susceptibility is a fingerprint of the pathogen. Arinaminpathy and McLean (2009) argue that adaptation driven by selection pressure in human hosts can play a significant role in allowing pathogens to cross the species barrier, as their mathematical model documents the potential markers of adaptation. Despite the unpredictability of infectious diseases and their adaptability for human transmission, their model suggests general patterns of behaviour that can be associated with different evolutionary pathways.

Because of the microbiological uncertainties and limited availability of data, the modelling and forecasting suffered from a lack of precise parameters. The severity of a pandemic is measured by estimates for the case: fatality rate, clinical attack rates and hospitalisation rates. The difficulties are acknowledged in the ECDC Pandemic Assessment Reports (Prevention 2009a):

> [On case : fatality rate] This is difficult to estimate with great accuracy at this stage and it should anyway be remembered that it is a measure that is sensitive to social factors (p. 11).

> [On clinical attack rate] In previous pandemics it was unusual to observe population clinical attack rates of less than 20%, while for seasonal influenza, rates are usually between 5% and 10%. However, this pandemic may be unusual since it seems that older people may be missing from those infected (pp. 9–10).

> [On hospitalisation rate] As this is a difficult to derive for Europe a rate observed from reported cases for the United States (11%) is correct but should not be used for planning, as it will be an overestimate (p. 11).

These contribute potential bias to estimates, according to Garske et al. (2009: 339s). The case : fatality ratio by definition is 'the ratio of the total number of deaths from a disease divided by the total number of cases'. Garske et al. (2009) note that estimating the case : fatality ratio works well in a fully ascertained epidemic, which is usually not the case. They argue that, for most infectious diseases, the number of cases cannot be fully confirmed. This is called 'underascertainment' because people who only have a mild infection or remain asymptomatic are not likely to seek health care and be tested. The reporting of the more severe cases that are diagnosed tends to overstate severity estimates.

Another source of bias arises when there is a delay between the disease onset and the final outcome in severe cases. This effect is called censoring and it means that the case : fatality ratio will remain low or will change (that is, grow) during the pandemic. These uncertainties are recognised by Lipsitch et al. (2009), who argue that two sources that critically affect severity estimates are the 'overestimation of the proportion of cases' and 'downward bias' because the estimates are calculated as simple ratios (Lipsitch et al. 2009: 113). What is common to these biases is a lack of observations and data, especially at the beginning of the pandemic. This lack of data was also mentioned in the early pandemic assessment model (Fraser et al. 2009). Moreover, these estimates are affected by variations in surveillance practices and national differences in pandemic policies. During the 2009 pandemic the UK decided to distribute antivirals (oseltamivir) on the basis of self-assessment whereas, in Finland, antivirals remained prescription medicines throughout the pandemic.

These uncertainties influence the projections that help characterise the pandemic. The stories that estimate the effectiveness of NPI or the effect of mitigation strategies embody uncertainties about behavioural assumptions and the model estimates, because their parameterisation uses data from the 1918 outbreak. The microbiological factors affect transmission and the future evolution of transmissibility, virulence and antiviral resistance bring uncertainty to the estimated predictions (Fraser et al. 2009). These uncertainties are acknowledged to be inbuilt limitations of the model, because they are based on the number of laboratory-confirmed cases and potential underestimations of morbidity. An increase in the availability of data may not be the only solution to reduce uncertainties in pandemic risk assessment. Limited knowledge of microbiological factors and difficulties in defining precise estimates affect the reliability of model-based evidence. It seems that the narratives, as necessary as they are to govern the pandemic, are able to provide only partial evidence for the governance of a pandemic.

Yet the early findings of severity and transmissibility, and estimates of how well mitigation strategies might work, turn into action plans and recommendations. The modelled narratives are capable of bringing together historical, social and epidemiological aspects and allow analyses of their effects both in the pre-pandemic and outbreak phases. Stories told by models are hardly ever complete and yet they gain authority over those who listen. To manage uncertainties that arise from incomplete and insufficient data sets and from the known and unknown factors that affect the course of a pandemic, modelling has proven to be a useful tool. When regarded as a technical rationality, modelling no longer appears as an innocent instrument but as a practice that embodies power relations. This is how modelling gains quantitative authority.

Towards narratives of governance

> Statistics help to create the reality they measure by providing a language for accessing it and techniques for its manipulation. (Espeland and Stevens 2008: 419)

Since the 2009 pandemic, its management has been questioned, both in the UK and globally. Was the pandemic alert unnecessary? Why did governments spend a significant amount of money on vaccinations and antiviral stocks, which have now expired? The story of the pandemic seems to remain partial. This was suggested when the UK government response was assessed in an independent report published in May 2010. This report discusses the use of modelling and its limitations as follows:

> In general, the early stages of what was to become the pandemic were characterised by uncertainty regarding various key parameters. Definitive scientific advice was therefore not always available. In a rapidly evolving situation, scientific decisions may be based on high levels of uncertainty, and this lack of certainty clearly frustrated ministers and policy officials at times. (Hine 2010: 66)

> Modelling also provides easily understandable figures, and because of its mathematical and academic nature may seem scientifically very robust. In light of this, it is understandable that ministers and officials set a great deal of store by modelling. (Hine, 2010: 67)

These observations confirm what we already learnt from the analysis of the models. Uncertainties were prevailing in the process, yet the persuasiveness of numbers made the models seem attractive and applicable to manage uncertainties:

> Early and emerging data should always be of some use, but its employment should be carefully managed. This is not to reject the use of models, but to understand its limitations: modellers are not 'court astrologers'. (Hine 2010: 67)

It seems that, despite their limitations, pandemic narratives become useful evidence for decision-making processes. It is easy to think that models yield firm and reliable evidence, although the risk assessment during the Swine flu pandemic pointed to the weak nature of evidence, due to unknown factors. The 2009 ECDC report assesses that 'the overall evidence is weak at present as it comes mostly from early observations of the pandemic and reported cases' (2009a: 3). This, as we learned from the built-in uncertainties, is often the case when a sudden, unpredicted event happens. Weak evidence sounds paradoxical: current policies consider an evidence base to be a strong and essential foundation for decision-making.

As quantifiable tools, models calculate and measure, but those 'mere' measurements also play a bigger role. They are tools that shape the object they measure and the social domain in which they are used. As Espeland and Stevens (2008: 419) argue, 'statistics help create reality they measure'. We can thus agree with Evans who argues that models are not 'truth machines' but a 'discursive space' that allows 'continuous dialogue' to shape understanding (Evans 2000: 223). Models can be seen as a form of technical rationality in the broader context of governmentality. As technical rationality, they become 'means, mechanisms, procedures, instruments, tactics, techniques, technologies and vocabularies' that constitute authority (Dean 2010: 42).

Despite the reported uncertainties, once the models deliver their results they gain an aura of authority. Why is that? This observation is not unique to models. It is, I suggest, part of the broader discourse of how numbers, numerical representations, measurement practices and processes of standardisation gain increasing authority and governance in current societies.

Acknowledgements

I would like to thank the British Academy Postdoctoral Fellowship and Research Fellowship with the Centre for Analysis of Risk and Regulation, LSE for financial support for this study. I thank the editors of this book and the two anonymous referees for constructive and insightful comments.

Notes

1   This estimate has been challenged by a recent model-based study that estimates the impact of the H1N1 pandemic outbreak on deaths from cardiovascular and respiratory diseases. Based on these estimates the H1N1 outbreak may have caused mortality rates that are 15 times higher than the laboratory-confirmed cases suggest (Dawood *et al.* 2012).
2   The basic reproductive rate, R_0, is determined by four factors: (i) the probability of transmission in a contact, (ii) the frequency of contacts, (iii) infectious period (of a person) and (iv) the proportion of immune in the population. (Giesecke 2002)

References

Arinaminpathy, N. and McLean, A. (2009) Evolution and emergence of novel human infections, *Proceedings of the Royal Society of London. Biological Sciences*, 276, 3937–43.
Balicer, R.D. (2007) Modeling infectious diseases dissemination through online role-playing games, *Epidemiology*, 18, 2, 260–1.
Bootsma, M.C.J. and Ferguson, N. (2007) The effect of public health measures on the 1918 influenza pandemic in U.S. cities, *PNAS*, 104, 18, 7588–93.
Dawood, F.S., Iuliani, A.D., Reed, C., Meltzer, M., *et al.* (2012) Estimated global mortality associated with the first 12 months of 2009 pandemic influenza A H1N1 virus circulation: a modelling study, *Lancet Infectious Diseases*, 12, 9, 687–95.
Dean, M. (2010) *Governmentality. Power and Rule in Modern Society*. London: Sage.

Department of Health (2010) Pandemic H1N1 vaccine uptake figures for England by SHA and PCT. Available at http://www.dh.gov.uk/en/Publicationsandstatistics/Publications/PublicationsPolicy AndGuidance/DH_114203 (accessed 15 August 2012).

Desrosières, A. (1998) *The Politics of Large Numbers: A History of Statistical Reasoning*. Cambridge: Harvard University Press.

den Butter, F. and Morgan, M. (2000) *Empirical Models and Policy-Making: Interaction and Institutions*. London: Routledge.

European Centre for Disease Control [ECDC] (2009a) Risk assessment report: pandemic (H1N1) 2009 influenza. 21 August. Stockholm. Available at http://ecdc.europa.eu/en/healthtopics/seasonal_influenza/assessments/pages/assessments.aspx (accessed 26 October 2012).

ECDC (2009a) Risk assessment report pandemic (H1N1) 2009 influenza. 25 September. Stockholm. Available at http://ecdc.europa.eu/en/healthtopics/seasonal_influenza/assessments/pages/assessments.aspx (accessed 26 October 2012).

ECDC (2009b) Risk assessment report pandemic (H1N1) 2009 influenza. 6 November. Stockholm. Available at http://ecdc.europa.eu/en/healthtopics/seasonal_influenza/assessments/pages/assessments.aspx (accessed 26 October 2012).

ECDC (2012) *Narcolepsy in Association with Pandemic Influenza Vaccination (a Multi-Country European Epidemiological Investigation)*. Stockholm: ECDC.

Giesecke, J. (2002) *Modern Infectious Disease Epidemiology*. London: Arnold.

Espeland Nelson, W. and Stevens, M. (2008) A sociology of quantification, *European Journal of Sociology*, 49, 3, 410–36.

Evans, R. (2000) Economic models and economic policy: what economic forecasts can do for government. In F. Butter, M. Morgan (eds) *Empirical Models and Policy-Making: Interaction and Institutions*. London: Routledge.

Ferguson, N.M., Cummings, D.A.T., Fraser, C., Cajka, J., *et al.* (2006) Strategies for mitigating an influenza pandemic, *Nature*, 442, 7101, 448–52.

Fox Keller, E. (2000) Models of and models for: theory and practice in contemporary biology, *Philosophy of Science*, 67, 3, S72–86.

Fox Keller, E. (2003) Experiments without material intervention. In H. Radder (ed.) *The Philosphy of Scientific Experimentation*, Pittsburgh: University of Pittsburgh Press.

Fraser, C., Donnelly, C.A., Cauchemez, S., Hanage, W., *et al.* (2009) Pandemic potential of a strain of influenza A (H1N1): early findings, *Science*, 324, 5934, 1557–61.

Garoon, J.P. and Duggan, P.S. (2008) Discourses of disease, discourses of disadvantage: a critical analysis of national pandemic influenza preparedness plans, *Social Science & Medicine*, 67, 7, 1133–42.

Garske, T., Legrand, J., Donnelly, C., Ward, H., *et al.* (2009) Assessing the severity of the novel influenza A/H1N1 pandemic, *British Medical Journal*, 339, doi: 10.1136/bmj.b2840.

Gerth, H.H. and Wright Mills, C. [1946](1958): *From Max Weber: Essays in Sociology*. Abingdon: Routledge.

Gramelsberger, G. (2010) Story telling with code. In A. Gleininger and G. Vrachliotis (eds) *Code. Between Operation and Narration*. Basel: Birkhauser.

Habbema, J.D., De Vlas, S.J., Plaisier, A.P. and Van Oortmarssen, G.J. (1996) The microsimulation approach to epidemiologic modeling of helminthic infections, with special reference to schistosomiasis, *American Journal of Tropical Medicine and Hygiene*, 55, 5 (Suppl), 165–9.

Hampton Frost, W. [1936](1965) Introduction. In J. Snow, *Snow on Cholera; being a Reprint of Two Papers*. New York: Hafner.

Hatchett, R., Mercher, C. and Lipstich, M. (2007) Public health interventions and epidemic intensity during the 1918 influenza pandemic, *Proceedings of the National Academy of Sciences USA*, 104, 18, 7582–7.

Hine, D.D. (2010) *The 2009 Influenza Pandemic. An Independent Review of the UK Response to the 2009 Influenza Pandemic*. London: Cabinet Office.

Institute for Health and Welfare (2011) National narcolepsy task force interim report. Helsinki, Institute for Health and Welfare. Available at http://www.thl.fi/thl-client/pdfs/dce182fb-651e-48a1-b018-3f774d6d1875 (accessed 1 October 2012).

Jasanoff, S. (ed.) (2004) *States of Knowledge: the Co-Production of Science and Social Order*. London: Routledge.

Landström, C., Whatmore, S.J. and Lane, S.N. (2011) Virtual engineering: computer simulation modelling for UK flood risk management, *Science Studies*, 24, 2, 3–22.

Latour, B. and Woolgar, S. [1979] (1986). *Laboratory Life: the Social Construction of Scientific Facts*. London: Sage.

Leach, M. and Dry, S. (2010) Epidemic narratives. In S. Dry and M. Leach (eds) *Epidemics. Science, Governance and Social Justice*. London: Earthscan.

Lipsitch, M., Riley, S., Cauchemez, S., Ghani, A., *et al.* (2009) Managing and reducing uncertainty in an emerging influenza pandemic, *New England Medical Journal*, 361, 2, 112–15.

Lofgren, E.T. and Fefferman, N. (2007) The untapped potential of virtual game worlds to shed light on real world epidemics, *The Lancet*, 7, 9, 625–9.

MacKenzie, D. (1990) *Inventing Accuracy. Historical Sociology of Nuclear Missile Guidance*. Cambridge: MIT Press.

Mansnerus, E. (2012) Understanding and governing public health risks by modeling. In S. Roeser, R. Hillerbrand, P. Sandin and M. Peterson (eds.) *Handbook of Risk Theory*. Dordrecht: Springer.

Merz, M. (1999) Multiplex and unfolding: computer simulation in particle physics, *Science in Context*, 12, 2, 293–316.

Morgan, M. (2001) Models, stories and the economic world, *Journal of Economic Methodology*, 8, 3, 361–84.

Morgan, M. (2012) *The World in the Model. How Economists Work and Think*. Cambridge: Cambridge University Press.

Morgan, M. and Morrison, M. (1999), *Models as Mediators. Perspectives on Natural and Social Sciences*. Cambridge: Cambridge University Press.

Nerlich, B. and Halliday, C. (2007) Avian flu: the creation of expectations between science and media, *Sociology of Health & Illness*, 29, 1, 46–65.

Nicoll, A. and Coulombier, D. (2009) Europe's initial experience with pandemic (H1N1) – mitigation and delaying policies and practices, *Euro Surveillance*, 14, 29.

Pinch, T. and Bijker, W. (1984) Social construction of facts and artefacts or how the sociology of science and sociology of technology might benefit each other, *Social Studies of Science*, 14, 3, 399–441.

Porter, T. (1995) *Trust in Numbers: the Pursuit of Objectivity in Science and Public Life*. Princeton: Princeton University Press.

Porter, T. (2000) Life insurance, medical testing and the management of mortality. In L. Daston (ed.) *Biographies of Scientific Objects*. Chicago: University of Chicago Press.

Power, M. (1997) *The Audit Society: Rituals of Verification*. Oxford: Clarendon Press.

Prior, L. (2006) Doing things with documents. In D. Silverman (ed.) *Qualitative Research. Theory, Method and Practice*. London: Sage.

Rudinow Saetnan, A., Mark Lomell, H. and Hammer, S. (2011) *The Mutual Construction of Statistics and Society*. London: Taylor and Francis.

Shackley, S. and Wynne, B. (1996) Representing uncertainty in global climate science and policy. Boundary-ordering devices and authority, *Science, Technology and Human Values*, 21, 3, 275–302.

Smith, R., Keogh-Brown, M. and Barnett, T. (2011) Estimating economic impact of pandemic influenza: an application of the computable general equilibrium model to the UK, *Social Science & Medicine*, 73, 2, 235–44.

Spiegelhalter, D. and Riesch, H. (2011) Don't know, can't know. Embracing deeper uncertainties when analysing risks, *Philosophical Transactions of the Royal Society A*, 369, 1956, 4730–50.

Stephenson, N. and Jamieson, M. (2009) Securitising health: Australian newspaper coverage of pandemic influenza, *Sociology of Health & Illness*, 31, 4, 525–39.

Stirling, A. and Scoones, I. (2009) From risk assessment to knowledge mapping: science, precaution and participation in disease ecology, *Ecology and Society*, 14, 2.

Strathern, M. (ed.) (2000) *Audit Cultures. Anthropological Studies in Accountability, Ethics and the Academy*. London: Routledge.

van Egmond, S. and Zeiss, R. (2010) Modelling for policy: science-based models as performative boundary objects for Dutch policy-making, *Science Studies*, 23, 1, 58–78.

Wallis, P. and Nerlich, B. (2005) Disease metaphors in the new epidemics: the UK media framing of the 2003 SARS epidemic, *Social Science & Medicine*, 60, 11, 2629–39.

World Health Organization (WHO) (2009) Global Alert and Response. No rationale for travel restrictions 1 May. Available at http://www.who.int/csr/disease/swineflu/guidance/public_health/travel_advice/en/index.html.

WHO (2011) Global alert and response (2011) Pandemic (H1N1) 2009 – update 100. Weekly update. Available at http://www.who.int/csr/disease/swineflu/laboratory14_05_2010/en/index.html (accessed 1 October 2012).

Wynne, B. (1992) Uncertainty and environmental learning. Reconceiving science and policy in the preventive paradigm, *Global Environmental Change*, 2, 2, 111–17.

Yearley, S. (1999) Computer models and the public's understanding of science: a case-study analysis, *Social Studies of Science*, 29, 6, 845–66.

11

Exploring the ambiguous consensus on public–private partnerships in collective risk preparation

Véronique Steyer and Claude Gilbert

Introduction

In France, the definition of the problem posed by the threat of an influenza pandemic has gradually incorporated the question of maintaining the fundamentals of social life. The potential length of such a crisis (three successive phases of 10–12 weeks, using Spanish flu as a benchmark), with part of the working population absent from their jobs due to illness or confinement, and disruptions in the supply of all types of goods and services, are reasons to fear an impairment or interruption of vital services (Gilbert *et al.* 2010). Consequently, the realisation that these services are part of a complex network of interdependencies has drawn attention to the question of the continuity of all organisational actors in the economy. Alongside public authorities, which tackled the issue in response to the World Health Organisation (WHO) alert (1999), it has gradually been recognised that other economic actors, especially companies, have a role in preparing for this 'major' risk, which like certain natural or technological risks (Lagadec 1981) may cause profound disturbances in modern societies.

Once considered potential sources of danger, generating industrial risks (Beck 1992, Perrow 1984), private-sector organisations, including companies, are now seen as indispensable partners in risk preparation and response. This shift, also observed for other types of risk (Borraz 2008), raises the question of the coordination between these different actors – coordination which is crucial to the effectiveness of the preparations (Dingwall 2008). The literature, especially that focusing on the question of public–private partnerships (PPPs) and inter-organisational collaborations, identifies numerous challenges (e.g. Greve and Hodge 2005, Huxham and Vangen 2000, Klijn and Teisman 2003).

This chapter analyses the conditions and difficulties of such a collaboration in preparing for a major collective risk. It is based on a study of the relations between French public authorities and companies before and during the alert raised by the 2009 outbreak of A(H1N1). The French case is particularly interesting because, spurred by public authorities, the country quickly undertook preparations to handle the flu pandemic threat (Mounier-Jack and Cooker 2006). The need to mobilise the private sector gradually became evident (Gilbert 2007) while a discourse on the necessity of a partnership between the various actors emerged.

Pandemics and Emerging Infectious Diseases: The Sociological Agenda, First Edition. Edited by Robert Dingwall, Lily M. Hoffman and Karen Staniland. Chapters © 2013 The Authors. Book Compilation © 2013 Foundation for the Sociology of Health & Illness / John Wiley & Sons Ltd.

The analysis shows, however, that, despite this assertion, the conditions necessary for a true 'partnership' were not achieved. Owing to various constraints and ambiguities, both public authorities and large companies took action on the flu pandemic (and other collective risks) within the framework of a poorly organised system, which itself is a risk factor. The study thus paints a more nuanced picture of the exhortation to set up PPPs to prepare for and manage collective risks and questions the desirability of this type of relationship in the specific context of risk management.

After tracing the evolving role of companies in the sociology of disasters, accidents and natural catastrophes, and discussing the difficulties of public–private collaboration evoked in the literature, we examine the possibilities and limitations of a PPP to manage the pandemic risk in the French context. We will conclude by exploring the impact of the ensuing reciprocal expectations effect on the country's preparation for these collective risks.

Companies: from 'risk-generator' to 'partner' in dealing with risks

In the sociology of disasters, accidents and natural catastrophes, companies are mainly studied from the angle of the dangers they generate. This is especially true of companies that employ dangerous technologies (nuclear, chemicals, etc.) or technologies whose effects are unknown (genetically modified organisms (GMOs), nanotechnologies, etc.). Numerous catastrophes have demonstrated the limitations of man's ability to control certain technologies (Zinn and Taylor-Gooby 2006), bolstering the argument that accidents are inevitable or even 'normal' in certain types of technological system (Perrow 1984). Controversies have arisen concerning 'new risks' that are harder to define, but which may eventually have equally catastrophic effects (Godard et al. 2002). Emphasis is placed on the negative effects on safety from economic pressures and production targets (Vaughan 1996). In this perspective, companies are seen less as producers of 'goods' than 'bads' (Beck and Holzner 2007: 10–11), contributing to the creation of a 'risk society' (Beck 1992).

Although quite dominant, this view has been qualified, however. Researchers have described the specific characteristics of high reliability organisations which, although they work with complex, high-risk technologies, have nevertheless managed to avoid accidents for long periods, while still attaining challenging production targets (Rochlin et al. 1987, La Porte 1988, Bourrier 1996). Although Weick (1987) has shown the difficulties of such an endeavour, research has lent support to the idea that managers can build resilient organisations (Sullivan-Taylor and Wilson 2009). These organisations are being held up as models to all companies confronted with uncertainty and a great deal of study is being done on the resilience of organisations (Hollnagel et al. 2006, Weick and Sutcliffe 2007, Comfort et al. 2010).

With the inevitability of catastrophes being challenged, a new approach to the role of companies is now possible. Companies are playing a key role in the management of high-risk activities by constantly working to ensure safety, which goes beyond compliance with the rules enacted by the public agencies that regulate these activities. Companies' capacity for autonomous risk management is now recognised. Added to this is the idea that they are also capable of mobilising precious competencies to deal with the aftermath of technological accidents (even where they bear no responsibility) as well as natural disasters and public health problems (Clarke 1999). The role to be played by companies in handling collective risks has therefore evolved. Companies – especially those involved in the production of goods and services or managing large networks (energy, transport, etc.) – are now also seen as indispensable partners in risk management. It is hardly surprising then that people are calling for the development of public–private collaborations to handle large-scale risks (Godard et al. 2002). The 'whole-of-society approach' has also gained acceptance internationally as the appropriate way of preparing for a pandemic threat (Ong et al. 2008).

Pessimistic literature on the potential of a public–private partnership (PPP)

This evolution raises the question of the coordination – crucial to the effectiveness of preparations – between these different actors (Dingwall 2008). What form might such a collaboration take?

The abundant literature on PPPs explores different formats in different contexts, with great variations and imprecision on the conceptual level (Brinkerhoff and Brinkerhoff 2011). At a minimum, PPPs can be defined as 'cooperative institutional arrangements between public and private sector actors' (Greve and Hodge 2005: 1). There are different PPP approaches depending on their goals, context and formal structures and the actors involved (Weihe 2008). Among these, we find the 'infrastructure approach', based on a contract with the public sector as principal and the private sector as agent, including the prior identification and allocation of risks (Bing et al. 2005). In contrast, the 'urban regeneration approach' emphasises co-production and risk sharing (Klijn and Teisman 2003) and envisages PPPs as a complex cooperation involving actors from different networks and spheres. Since public and private sectors operate with different norms, procedures and values, they are hard to reconcile (e.g. Jacobs 1992). Opting for a more flexible framework, the 'policy approach' sees the PPP as constellations of public and private actors arranged around a specific domain (Vaillancourt Roseneau 2000, Weihe 2008). It may even be conceived of as a specific form of governance, a non-hierarchical coordination different from the two conventional forms (market and hierarchy). It is no longer a question of dividing responsibilities, but of pluralist representation and transparency in policy-making (Börzel 1998).

This variety implies that partners' expectations as to the nature of their cooperation may diverge, thus engendering a disconcerting ambiguity. There may also be additional difficulties that are common to every inter-organisational collaboration. Membership is often a source of ambiguity (Huxham and Vangen 2000): its scope is vague, relations between individual and organisational members are uncertain, and numerous partnerships with overlapping membership are a source of complexity. Each organisation's constraints and the internal tensions between collaboration and competition may compromise the reliability of individuals' commitments (Babiak and Thibault 2009). Collaboration is a dynamic, emergent and non-linear process (Thompson and Perry 2006). External pressure and shifting goals cause its structure to change constantly. These dynamics and complexities make it hard to build relations of trust (Huxham and Vangen 2000, Huxham 2003). Yet trust is an important if not an indispensable factor for success (Ostrom 1998, Faulkner and de Rond 2000), though it is rarely present initially. Thanks to reputation, experience and formal contracts, partners can take the risk of diving in and thus initiating a trust-building loop (Vangen and Huxham 2003). Expensive and arduous, collaboration can easily lead to 'collaborative inertia' (Huxham 2003).

In risk management, issues of legitimacy and responsibility make relationships even more complex. In France, the preservation of public safety is a state prerogative. Through its core functions, known as 'fonctions régaliennes' (national defence, justice, police, etc.), the power of the state is affirmed (Gilbert 1992). This affirmation of authority and competence in public discourse is, however, often accompanied in practice by a certain disengagement of responsibility by public authorities (Borraz and Gilbert 2008). Responsibility is partly transferred to the organisations, mainly companies, that actually implement safety initiatives. But there are numerous ambiguities that tend to deter companies from taking on responsibility. Companies are more inclined to respond to directives from public authorities within the established regulatory framework (cf. requisitions), while endeavouring to solve their own difficulties, than to take initiatives and collaborate voluntarily in the prevention of collective risks. In each case, these initiatives are determined by company size and the extent of their network: there is a significant difference between large, medium and small companies.

Certain factors may, however, impel companies to be proactive. This is true of large companies, especially those involved in international trade. Seen as essentially determined by global market forces and somewhat insensitive to local concerns, multinationals often lack legitimacy (Beck and Holzner 2007). Getting involved in public health matters – undeniably a common good – through pandemic threat preparations can be a response to these growing criticisms (Herrick 2008). Additionally, this demonstration that they are 'good citizens' might bolster the social importance of their role as producers of indispensable goods and services for society. However, the public health (or environmental) efforts of these companies sometimes amount to no more than symbolic actions, like 'fantasy planning' (Clarke 1999), without any concrete impact. Offsetting the view of organisations as risk generators, the idea has emerged that good corporate governance has to include formalised risk management practices (Scheytt *et al.* 2006), which has stimulated the development of risk management systems (Power 2004) and the normalisation of business continuity management – a kind of crisis management focusing on resilience in the face of external shocks (Herbane 2010).

Studies on disasters, accidents and natural catastrophes tend to conclude that it is necessary to develop PPPs to manage collective risks. The spread of business continuity management practices may encourage companies, especially the largest ones, to go beyond mere window-dressing in these matters. Nevertheless, according to the literature on inter-organisational collaborations and PPPs, such collaborations face numerous challenges. How do these different movements mesh in practice? To answer this question, we will examine what happened in a particular case where a PPP was set up to face a collective risk: the flu pandemic in France.

Methods and data

The aim was to explore the different dimensions of public–private relationships in preparing a country for a collective risk. We chose the case study method to capture the interaction between the different movements identified in the literature and focused on a single case in order to examine its complexity in detail. We carried out interviews and used field observation to gather actors' discourses, representations and practices.

The first data-gathering phase, on preparations for an avian flu pandemic (A(H5N1) virus), was carried out between May and December 2008. We interviewed representatives from the business world (business continuity managers (BCMs), consultants and representatives of professional associations) and public authorities (government ministries, defence zones[1]). The sample was designed to collect the main actors' perceptions (purposive sample). Four representatives from companies and the governmental sphere were contacted. The sample was then expanded through a 'snowball' effect: public authorities' representatives gave contact names in companies, and vice versa. Four more people were approached independently to diversify affiliation networks and business sectors (state-owned companies, former state companies, private sector and subsidiaries of foreign companies). Altogether, 14 representatives from the business world and six from public authorities were interviewed. We also observed a conference on national preparation in September 2008 and a meeting in March 2009 where a group of BCMs in charge of flu pandemic preparations at their companies met to share their practices.

The A(H1N1) outbreak in April 2009 triggered a second stage of investigation where the main method used was observation. Ten BCM exchange-group meetings were observed between April 2009 and March 2010, and a national conference in September 2009. In addition, two public officials and three company representatives were re-interviewed and five new representatives from companies were approached.

The 30 interviews focused on large companies and national public authorities. This bias is a reflection of the groups most active in preparations, but was offset by observations (conferences, BCM groups) which involved a wider variety of actors (small and medium-sized enterprises (SMEs), associations, local government). The study probes the relations between national public authorities and large companies – actors focused on in the existing literature – and outlines the 'grey areas' between them and the other actors who may potentially be involved in flu pandemic preparation.

The interviews were semi-structured, lasting between 26 minutes and 4 hours (averaging 76 minutes). All were recorded and fully transcribed, except six (due to refusals or technical difficulties). For those, extensive notes were taken during the interview and completed immediately afterward. The same procedure was followed for the meetings. We acquired the minutes of the conferences and complemented them with notes taken by one of the authors. These texts were examined to identify any themes that emerged, with a view to describing and categorising the relations between public and private actors. These themes were then used to code and organise extracts of relevant data. When necessary, they were completed and modified during the coding process. We were careful to verify that the information from interviews with different types of respondent was consistent with naturally occurring data.

French preparation for the pandemic

Recognition by public authorities of the need to involve companies
Although the first version of the French pandemic response plan (2004) emphasised the public health issue and sought solutions from the perspective of a 'state of emergency', the anticipated length of the crisis gradually caused public authorities to consider the continuity of the country's vital infrastructures and the effects of a long crisis on the basic structures of society. Though incomplete, this shift was prompted by both internal government discussions and seminars that brought public officials and researchers together (Gilbert 2007, 2010). At the request of their corresponding ministries, a small number of large, private-sector and state-owned companies recognised as national critical infrastructure operators (CIOs) tackled the issue.

These companies disclosed their complex dependencies with respect to the national and international economic fabric. Employee absenteeism, procurement difficulties and monetary problems could combine and affect the country's economic and social functioning. While this may impair the ability to respond to the health issue, more broadly it jeopardises the ability to keep the economy running. The involvement of these CIOs prompted an exploration of the system's vulnerabilities. In the pandemic threat, the economic continuity problem is interwoven with the health problem. Companies are doubly concerned: they are both places of potential contamination and essential partners in the country's resilience.

The necessary 'partnership' discourse

The public officials in charge of the issue were now faced with the question of how to mobilise the private sector. An authoritarian approach would be at odds with the general tendency in France toward less government involvement. Most importantly, measures would be ineffective without the cooperation of companies, especially given the question of competency: 'asking the government to guide large or small companies in preparing business continuity plans (BCPs) would be a mistake' (public official, 2008).

The idea of a necessary shift in the governance of risks and crises took root in public authorities: '[The public officials in charge] have to work through recommendations, certifications, advice and partnerships' (public official, 2008). The partnership idea raises the question of how a public service mentality and a market mentality might work together: hybridisation, public service delegations to companies in times of crisis . . . how could it be done? (Gilbert 2007).

This partnership discourse found an echo in companies: 'This matter is a prime example of where we must become more involved in the principle of . . . public–private partnership' (employers' union, conference, 2008).

Ambiguous implementation

The scope of the partnership called for in discourses was hard to define. First, which 'public sector' and which 'private sector' were we talking about?

Many governmental actors were concerned: the inter-ministerial delegate to the fight against the influenza pandemic (DILGA), government ministries (health, economy, etc.), and so on. This issue required a high level of cooperation between ministries. But 'the interministerial aspect has always caused problems and continues to do so . . . [each ministry has] its own culture, strategy and very specific organisation' (public official, 2008). Moreover, the structures that would have to implement this 'inter-ministeriality' lacked the legitimacy to impose their will or they appeared to be precarious or even ambiguous (e.g. the DILGA only has a very small team, placed at his disposal temporarily). Assigning tasks was problematic: who, for example, should specify the roles to be played by companies? 'It could be the [Ministry of the Economy] acting with regard to companies in general. But other ministries might also lay claim to this function, such as the Labour Ministry' (public official, 2008). This complexity was disconcerting for companies as they lacked a clearly identified contact for pandemic preparations.

The companies were no more uniform, however, either in size or in their relations with public authorities. At first glance, it seemed easy to establish relations with large companies (those that operate internationally and those that were once – or remain partly – state-owned), especially as many of them – CIOs – are obliged to ensure the continuity of their activities. But this apparent ease of contact must be qualified: some companies openly 'reminded the government that their objective . . . is to make short term profits' (BCM of a privatised company, 2008). SMEs were even harder to reach. The actors usually in contact with them are not those in charge of pandemic preparations.

Finally, 'public' and 'private' are two spheres with different mentalities: 'the public sector often considers the private as this horrible little capitalist . . . and the private sector sees the public sector as . . . you just shrug your shoulders' (BCM, 2008). Each functions with a simplified vision of the other: the 'government' for companies and a focus on a few large companies for public authorities. In practice, the dialogue is engaged (or becomes strained) between the DILGA, the Ministries of the Economy and Labour on the public side and, on the company side, the largest, recognised CIOs, through a few professional associations and unions (Médef and industry unions).

Concretely, the way the government deals with companies remains fragmented, essentially based on individual initiatives (involvement in conferences, etc.). The national plan nevertheless anticipates more systematic integration of large companies in the subcommittees of the economic continuity taskforce, which would direct the country's economy in the event of a crisis.

Public appeals and the manifest willingness to form partnerships have, nevertheless, opened a space for dialogue, allowing selected companies to (attempt to) negotiate the details of the national plan. When confronted with a plan that called for the suspension of some of its activities, one company reaffirmed its necessity at a meeting and suggested a different way to plan for downgraded operations, better suited to the company's interests.

Finally, the appearance of new actors – BCMs – provides public authorities with a contact in companies to disseminate the business continuity subject. This ties in with the movement to normalise business continuity management (Herbane 2010). While it is more pronounced in English-speaking countries, and therefore in some French subsidiaries of American and British companies, large French companies with international operations are receptive, especially as discussions at French and European levels on the resilience of vital infrastructures have resulted in a business continuity obligation for CIOs in France (Secteurs d'Activités d'Importance Vitale (SAIV) decree, 2006). In this context, these BCMs are seeking a positioning closer to top management and a broader jurisdiction (Abbott 1988). Various professional associations are developing (though not without ambiguities: some of them are associated with consulting firms, others with international certification bodies) in which representatives from competing companies form alliances and exchange ideas while being careful not to reveal their vulnerabilities (excessively). Described as 'a bustling milieu that tries to take control of new ideas and "kill off" its neighbour' (consultant, 2008), these associations constitute competing interfaces between public authorities and companies. The pandemic is seen as a precedent-setting case, where the form its management takes will prefigure future regulations. For these BCMs, being part of these public–private networks is crucial and they are eager to have discussions with the public officials in charge of the issue.

Although determining the form of the partnership was problematic, initiatives and meeting places did develop. However, these initiatives were championed by individuals holding peripheral positions in their organisation. The search for external partners was therefore tied to an effort to consolidate their positions and build on this boundary-spanning role that echoes the 'marginal-secant' position described by Crozier and Friedberg (1977).

A major difficulty: assigning responsibilities

The partnership discourse is at odds with traditional (more central) positions and habitual modes of action, i.e. the affirmation of the central role of government in managing collective risks, with companies reduced to 'private operators having to implement [the plan]' (public official, conference, 2008). In keeping with this traditional view, the governmental mobilisation of companies apparently was largely done through labour and CIO regulations. Ultimately, the officially adopted recommendation stance appears limited. This recourse to the regulatory approach reignited issues of responsibility in the event of failure.

The opinions expressed by the interviewees on certain points reveal this entrenchment of positions. The idea that it fell to major corporations to spread the word about economic continuity was ill-received: 'We're not going to step in and do the authorities' job of explaining how to make a BCP . . . It's like the sword of Damocles . . .' (BCM, 2009). Similarly, the authorities' emphasis on business owners' legal obligation to guarantee the health and safety of their employees – and to produce results – came under fire; influenza is not a risk that is confined to companies. Some BCMs decried attempts to make companies shoulder responsibilities that exceeded their powers: obligations concerning employee safety transferred costs and responsibility to companies. Mask purchases became the symbol of a company's preparation, of compliance with regulations: 'The masks are wrapped up with the issue of the company's civil responsibility' (BCM, 2009).

Relations between public and private sector actors vis-à-vis the pandemic seem therefore to be strongly shaped by questions relating to the future attribution of responsibility. Everyone is careful not to go beyond their obligations.

The partnership discourse: complications rather than help in time of crisis?
These relations were tested by the outbreak of A(H1N1) in April 2009. The partnership discourse led some BCMs to expect that there would be more sharing. They were disappointed: large companies did not get more information than the general public and their participation in subgroups of the Economy Ministry's economic continuity taskforce turned out to be a one-way street. Although the partnership discourse did not live up to its promises, the affirmation of the government's central role led people to expect, at the very least, clear directives. But no strong message was forthcoming. No official position was announced on a coordinated signal to trigger the BCPs, in spite of the discussions on a new type of coordination between public authorities and civil society on risk preparation (Mallet *et al.* 2008). Further, the alert caused a change in the people in charge within the public authorities. When the crisis came, ministers' cabinets took over. For their contacts, 'it was very worrying, really quite distressing. The official contacts were just becoming familiar with the issue and didn't have any answers' (BCM, 2009).

In the eyes of the BCMs, the public authorities were not assuming their leadership role, nor were they entering the promised partnership. On the contrary, tensions were growing, owing to the anticipated transfer of responsibility. For example, the market supply of masks dried up due to government orders, provoking the ire of companies, which found themselves physically unable to comply with legislation. Any divergence by public authorities from their initial plan was seen as a betrayal by certain companies, especially by the BCMs who found themselves in an awkward position vis-à-vis their superiors. In short, relations between public authorities and large companies suffered from the lack of stabilised agreements and continuity in the system and interaction of actors.

Some large companies made direct contact with public officials locally. Rather than wait for answers 'from above', their BCMs handled concrete situations pragmatically, e.g. by having people wear masks when flu cases were detected. It was a lesson in forced autonomy: 'We were sent back to our companies to assess the risk. We were not to expect governmental instructions. But we were expected to take appropriate measures' (BCM, 2009).

The partnership discourse proclaimed by public authorities thus had harmful effects. The divergence between discourse and practices impaired the trust between participants and weakened their coordination, instead of improving it, though it is true that companies moved closer to local actors. Perhaps the readjustment was necessary, demonstrating the difficulty of managing a pandemic risk at a global level when the phenomenon is first and foremost local and growing unevenly in space and time. Doubt is cast on the role of national public authorities in managing this type of risk, however.

Ultimately, this episode sets a precedent in public–private relations for risk management. The disappointment experienced is not conducive to building trust between public and private actors which, according to many scholars, is crucial to the development of the sought-after partnership.

Discussion and conclusion

The research on disasters, accidents and natural catastrophes tends to conclude that PPPs should be developed to manage collective risks. Yet, numerous challenges have been identified in the literature on inter-organisational collaborations and PPPs. How do these movements interact in practice? To answer this question, we have analysed a particular case where PPPs were set up to face a collective risk: that of a flu pandemic in France.

This case highlights the difficulty public authorities and large companies had in positioning themselves. Although both sides seemed to recognise the necessity of partnership, many obstacles arose, echoing the literature: different cultures and modes of operation (Jacobs 1992); multiple arenas engendering problems marking out boundaries (Klijn and Teisman 2003); and ambiguity concerning the nature, scope and membership of the partnership (Huxham and Vangen 2000). The difficulties of adapting to a new type of relationship, with each actor retreating to familiar modes of action (regulation and contractual allocation of responsibilities) (Klijn and Teisman 2003), resulted in anticipated transfers of responsibility and reciprocal expectations effect.

Moreover, the case shows that the particularities of the domain (collective risk preparation and management) dealt with by this partnership placed the actors within a system that was particularly impacted by the anticipation of socio-political or 'secondary' risks (legal, reputation, individual blame) (Power 2004). This system weakened their positions, especially as they were often peripheral actors trying simultaneously to promote their ideas while strengthening their legitimacy within their own organisations. In this situation, the divergence observed between the 'partnership' discourse and practices during the A(H1N1) alert appears to be both the product of a poorly organised system and a force that perpetuates the system, as it impairs the trust between actors and weakens their coordination rather than improving it. Together with the difficulties commonly found in inter-organisational collaborations and partnerships, this poorly organised system is evidence of the need for a more nuanced picture of PPP development to prepare for and manage collective risks.

More precisely, one may wonder whether 'partnership' is a suitable term for such a relationship. Although there is no sharing of responsibilities, we do observe a kind of 'co-production' in formulating the pandemic plan. The many discussions between representatives of public authorities and companies may indicate the emergence of a 'policy PPP' (Börzel 1998). The obstacles arise in moving from the formulation of the plan to its implementation, and intensify when a reconfiguration is necessary to manage a specific project: the A(H1N1) outbreak. Although the policy PPP does not broach the question of risk-sharing – only the government can bear responsibility for policy in a democratic regime (Börzel 1998) – this transition demands action from companies. Either this action is done to comply with a regulatory obligation (and the BCMs can hide behind the public decision), or it is the result of acknowledged co-production and leads to responsibility sharing.

What is striking is that neither party seems to want to establish a more formal partnership, preferring to maintain ambiguities in their relationship. Paradoxically, although the

BCMs seem to be spear-heading the response to the pandemic risk in their companies, they also constitute a barrier to the modification of the relationship formed between companies and public authorities. Their position does not favour the idea of co-production and shared responsibility. Although the data do not allow one to judge the extent of all the companies' preparations, certain companies carried out actions that went far beyond mere window-dressing. One factor determining their actions (mask purchases, formulation of plans) is undeniably the goal of compliance. The BCMs were angered when they found it impossible for them to comply, owing to contradictory directives from authorities. One may then question the true nature of the risk managed by companies. Are they managing the pandemic risk at the primary level, or 'secondary', individual and organisational risks (Power 2004)?

By extension, a more pronounced formalisation of the partnership would raise the question of accountability. Paradoxically, in becoming partners in the management of societal risks, companies would, rather than shoring up their faltering legitimacy (Beck and Holzner 2007), run the risk of weakening it further as they would be compelled to take eminently political decisions without being democratically mandated to do so. What then might be the legitimate place of a company – a non-elected actor – in decisions relating to societal risks in a democratic regime? Is such a formalisation really in companies' interests?

Likewise, for public authorities, relinquishing the prerogative of protecting the population would undermine a founding element of their role and mission. While large companies can do more than they say and the government says more than it can do, the relationship between these two spheres seems to hang on ambiguities that are best not clarified. Moreover, if public authorities were to engage in a true partnership (with co-production and shared responsibility), would they be able to justify the role they assign to the companies selected? Here we find the legitimacy problem of policy PPPs in democratic regimes, which threatens the effectiveness of the very policies they support (Börzel 1998). The formalisation of a policy PPP for risk management would be subjected to extreme vigilance and any mistake could easily spark a scandal.

Acknowledgements

This research project benefited from the support of the Fondation pour une Culture de Sécurité Industrielle (Foundation for an Industrial Safety Culture) and the 'Risk Strategy and Performance' Chair of ESCP Europe/KPMG. The authors gratefully acknowledge the insightful comments of Robert Dingwall and two anonymous reviewers. They thank Hervé Laroche, Jean-Philippe Bouilloud and Loizos Heracleous for helpful comments and suggestions on drafts of this work.

Note

1   Defence zones are administrative districts in charge of organising the civil and economic defence of the country.

References

Abbott, A. (1988) *The System of Professions: An Essay on the Division of Expert Labor*. Chicago, IL: University of Chicago Press.

Babiak, K. and Thibault, L. (2009) Challenges in multiple cross-sector partnerships, *Nonprofit and Voluntary Sector Quarterly*, 38, 1, 117–43.

Beck, U. (1992) *Risk Society: Towards a New Modernity*. London: Sage.

Beck, U. and Holzner, B. (2007) Organizations in world risk society. In Pearson, C.M., Roux-Dufort, C. and Clair, J.A. (eds) *International Handbook of Organizational Crisis Management*. Thousand Oaks, CA: Sage.

Bing, L., Akintoye, A., Edwards, P. and Hardcastle, C. (2005) The allocation of risks in PPP/PFI construction projects in the UK, *International Journal of Project Management*, 23, 1, 25–35.

Borraz, O. (2008) *Les politiques du risque*. Paris: Presse de Sciences Po.

Borraz, O. and Gilbert, C. (2008) Quand l'Etat prend des risques. In Borraz, O. and Guiraudon, V. (eds) *Politiques publiques 1. La France dans la gouvernance européenne*. Paris: Presses de Sciences Po.

Börzel, T.A. (1998) Organizing Babylon – on the different conceptions of policy networks, *Public Administration*, 76, 2, 253–73.

Bourrier, M. (1996) Organizing maintenance work at two American nuclear power plants, *Journal of Contingencies and Crisis Management*, 4, 2, 104–12.

Brinkerhoff, D.W. and Brinkerhoff, J.M. (2011) Public–private partnerships: perspectives on purposes, publicness, and good governance, *Public Administration and Development*, 31, 1, 2–14.

Clarke, L. (1999) *Mission Improbable, Using Fantasy Documents to Tame Disaster*. Chicago, IL: University of Chicago Press.

Comfort, L.K., Boin, A. and Demchak, C. (eds) (2010) *Designing Resilience: Preparing for Extreme Events*. Pittsburgh, PA: University of Pittsburgh Press.

Crozier, M. and Friedberg, E. (1977) *L'acteur et le système*. Paris: du Seuil.

Dingwall, R. (2008) Pandemic influenza – a social science perspective. In 1st International Workshop on Ethical Issues in European National Preparedness for Pandemic Influenza, 20–21 November 2008. Paris: AP-HP.

Faulkner, O. and de Rond, M. (2000) Perspectives on cooperative strategy. In Faulkner, O. and de Rond, M. (eds) *Corporate Strategy*. Oxford: Oxford University Press.

Gilbert, C. (1992) *Le pouvoir en situation extrême. Catastrophes et Politique*. Paris: L'Harmattan.

Gilbert, C. (ed.) (2007) *Les crises sanitaires de grande ampleur: un nouveau défi?* Paris: La Documentation française.

Gilbert, C. (2010) Policies and plans for long-term crisis management: the case of avian flu. In Boin, A., Comfort, L. and Demchak, C. (eds) *Designing Resilience for Extreme Events: Sociotechnical Approaches*. Pittsburgh, PA: Pittsburgh University Press.

Gilbert, C., Bourdeaux, I. and Raphaël, L. (2010) La résilience, un enjeu politique? L'approche française du risque de pandémie grippale (H5N1), *Télescope*, 16, 2, 22–36.

Godard, O., Henry, C., Lagadec, P. and Michel-Kerjan, E. (2002) *Traité des nouveaux risques – Précaution, Crise, Assurance*. Paris: Gallimard.

Greve, C. and Hodge, G. (2005) Introduction. In Hodge, G. and Greve, C. (eds) *The Challenge of Public–Private Partnerships: Learning from International Evidence*. Cheltenham: Edward Elgar.

Herbane, B. (2010) The evolution of business continuity management: a historical review of practices and drivers, *Business History*, 52, 6, 978–1002.

Herrick, C. (2008) Shifting blame/selling health: corporate social responsibility in the age of obesity, *Sociology of Health and Illness*, 31, 1, 51–65.

Hollnagel, E., Woods, D.D. and Leveson, N. (eds) (2006) *Resilience Engineering: Concepts and Precepts*. Aldershot UK and Burlington VT: Ashgate.

Huxham, C. (2003) Theorizing collaboration practice, *Public Management Review*, 5, 3, 401–23.

Huxham, C. and Vangen, S. (2000) Ambiguity, complexity and dynamics in the membership of collaboration, *Human Relations*, 53, 6, 771–806.

Jacobs, J. (1992) *Systems of Survival: A Dialogue on the Moral Foundations of Commerce and Politics*. Mississauga, OT: Random House.

Klijn, E.H. and Teisman, G.R. (2003) Institutional and strategic barriers to public–private partnership: an analysis of Dutch cases, *Public Money and Management*, 23, 3, 137–46.

La Porte, T.R. (1988) The United States air traffic system: increasing reliability in the midst of rapid growth. In Mayntz, R. and Hughes, T. (eds) *The Development of Large Scale Systems*. Boulder, CO: Westview.

Lagadec, P. (1981) *La civilisation du risque: catastrophes technologiques et responsabilité sociale*. Paris: du Seuil.

Mallet, J.-C., Présidence de la République (France) et Ministè re de la défense (France) (2008) *Défense et Sécurité nationale: le Livre blanc*. Paris: La Documentation française.

Mounier-Jack, S. and Coker, R.J. (2006) How prepared is Europe for pandemic influenza? Analysis of national plans, *Lancet*, 367, 9520, 1405–11.

Ong, A., Kindhauser, M., Smith, I. and Chan, M. (2008) A global perspective on avian influenza, *Annals of the Academy of Medicine Singapore*, 37, 477–81.

Ostrom, E. (1998) A behavioral approach to the rational choice theory of collective action. *American Political Science Review*, 92, 1, 1–23.

Perrow, C. (1984) *Normal Accidents: Living with High-Risk Technologies*. New York, NY: Basic.

Power, M. (2004) *The Risk Management of Everything: Rethinking the Politics of Uncertainty*. London: DEMOS.

Rochlin, G.I., La Porte, T.R. and Roberts, K.H. (1987) The self-designing high-reliability organization: aircraft carrier operations at sea, *Naval War College Review*, 40, 76–90.

Scheytt, T., Soin, K., Sahlin-Andersson, K. and Power, M. (2006) Introduction: Organizations, risk and regulation, *Journal of Management Studies*, 43, 6, 1331–7.

Sullivan-Taylor, B. and Wilson, D.C. (2009) Managing the threat of terrorism in British travel and leisure organizations, *Organization Studies*, 30, 2–3, 251–76.

Thompson, A.M. and Perry, J. (2006) Collaboration processes: inside the black box, *Public Administration Review*, 66, s1, 34–43.

Vaillancourt Roseneau, P. (ed.) (2000) *Public–Private Policy Partnerships*. Cambridge, MA: MIT Press.

Vangen, S. and Huxham, C. (2003) Nurturing collaborative relations: building trust in inter-organizational collaboration, *Journal of Applied Behavioral Science*, 39, 1, 5–31.

Vaughan, D. (1996) *The Challenger Launch Decision*. Chicago, IL: University of Chicago Press.

Weick, K.E. (1987) Organizational culture as a source of high reliability, *California Management Review*, 29, 112–27.

Weick, K.E. and Sutcliffe, K.M. (2007) *Managing the Unexpected: Resilient Performance in the Age of the Uncertainty*, 2nd edn. San Francisco, CA: Wiley.

Weihe, G. (2008) Ordering disorder – on the perplexities of the partnership literature, *Australian Journal of Public Administration*, 67, 4, 430–42.

Zinn, J.O. and Taylor-Gooby, P.F. (2006) Risk as an interdisciplinary research area. In Taylor-Gooby, P.F. and Zinn, J.O. (eds) *Risk in Social Science*. Oxford: Oxford University Press.

12

'If you have a soul, you will volunteer at once': gendered expectations of duty to care during pandemics
Rebecca Godderis and Kate Rossiter

Contemporary public health crises, such as influenza A virus subtype H1N1 and severe acute respiratory syndrome, have illuminated the complicated issues that arise in relation to the social and ethical dilemmas inherent in pandemic planning. In particular, the duty to care, defined in current day contexts as the professional rights and responsibilities of healthcare providers, has been identified as a pressing ethical issue. However, nuanced discussions of the nature of duty to care are relatively limited in contemporary debates about pandemic preparedness (Joint Centre for Bioethics Pandemic Ethics Working Group 2008). Given that healthcare providers are exposed to greater levels of risk in terms of both morbidity and mortality during outbreaks of mass infectious disease, it is critical to understand the interchange between moral or ethical obligation (that is, the socially constructed imperatives) and physical risk. In this chapter we argue that increased risk during a pandemic is an issue that is at once moral and gendered, and thus uniquely social in its orientation.

We explore this dimension of pandemic risk by using a socio-historical perspective – a particularly productive mechanism for shedding light on potential social and ethical concerns in the current context. Using a socio-historical lens allows us to identify patterns that may be replicated in contemporary society but can be difficult to recognise, given our collective embeddedness in the present day. Specifically, our empirical data point to the moral and gendered nature of duty to care during the 1918 influenza pandemic, and thus we argue that these findings should encourage pandemic planners to reflect on how such dynamics may pertain to, and indeed replicate themselves in, contemporary healthcare settings. These findings are particularly important in the face of potential emergent pandemics. While it is commonly believed that the current context of healthcare work is distinct from the early 20th century, in fact most front-line healthcare providers continue to be women (Adams 2010) and it is front-line workers who face disproportionate risks of illness and death during a pandemic (Ruderman *et al.* 2006).

Our historical research on the moral and gendered dimensions of pandemic risk documented the experience of the Canadian city of Brantford, Ontario during the 1918 influenza pandemic. Brantford was chosen as the site for analysis because it suffered very high rates of infection during the pandemic. Further, Brantford was a thriving and highly populated, multicultural industrial centre during the early 20th century, which means that its experience of the pandemic was well documented in public records. Archival material was collected from Brantford City Hall, local newspapers, the local Board of Trade and the nursing school

Pandemics and Emerging Infectious Diseases: The Sociological Agenda, First Edition. Edited by Robert Dingwall, Lily M. Hoffman and Karen Staniland. Chapters © 2013 The Authors. Book Compilation © 2013 Foundation for the Sociology of Health & Illness / John Wiley & Sons Ltd.

at the Brantford General Hospital. Newspaper articles from the city's two major dailies, *The Expositor and the Courier*, are the key source of empirical data used in this chapter. However, our results are informed by a broad reading of all primary data sources. Content analysis of textual sources indicates that expectations about duty to care during the 1918 pandemic were gendered in three specific ways: (i) presumptions about women's innate caregiving skills, (ii) moral claims about women's obligation to provide care and (iii) a lack of recognition of women's work and authority. We argue that this particular construction of the duty to care placed women at a greater risk for pandemic-related illness.

In her history of Canadian nursing practice McPherson (1996: 15) notes that the nursing profession has always been guided by the gendered assumption that 'personal service tasks demanded in patient care were deemed natural for women to execute'. Evidence from the archival record indicates that this belief informed expectations of the duty to care in Brantford during the 1918 influenza pandemic, resulting in city leaders appealing to all female community members to volunteer as nurses to look after the ill. Otherwise stated, in this particular socio-historical context the notion of duty to care extended beyond the boundaries of professionally trained caregivers and into the lay population where it assumed a gendered nature. Newspaper articles report on meetings between city councillors and the Board of Health in which male leaders of the community argue that if even 'two or three trained nurses could be secured, volunteers could do the remainder of the work' (*The Expositor* 1918a: 1), suggesting that the kind of work required in nursing would simply come naturally to those who volunteered. Moreover, once the schools closed all teachers, over 85% of whom were women,[1] were strongly encouraged by the Chairman of the Board of Education to volunteer as nurses until the schools re-opened. Similar requests were not made for other (presumably male) citizens who were unable to work due to a city declaration that all churches, theatres and other 'places of amusement' be closed (*Courier* 1918a: 1).

In her work on the impact of the 1918 influenza pandemic in Winnipeg, Manitoba Jones (2008) documents a similar trend, noting that public appeals to volunteer were directed almost exclusively at women and were based on a gendered assumption about their innate caregiving abilities. Moreover, Jones argues this assumption trumped any actual nursing ability: the call for volunteer nurses continued in spite of the fact that trained nurses reported that untrained volunteers were unable to make significant contributions because they did not know what to do.[2] Similarly, in Brantford comments made by Mr C.G. Ellis, member of the Board of Health, illustrate how gender, the duty to care and caregiving skills were assumed to be linked:

> I think the women will respond to an appeal for volunteer nurses. There must be hundreds in Brantford who have had experience, and many others who know a little about the work. *Courier* (1918b: 6)

Despite gendered assumptions of caregiving ability, the volunteers' actual abilities to nurse became a cause for concern (*Courier* 1918b: 6). In an attempt to mitigate the tension caused by the difference between women's perceived and actual caregiving ability, a teacher from a medical college in Toronto, Ontario, Mr Stoker, was brought to Brantford to provide basic training to volunteer nurses, such as how to apply mustard plasters, poultices and cold packs. To reach the largest number of potential volunteers, this information was also reprinted in detail in *The Expositor* (1918b: 5). Thus, despite the commonly held belief that any female volunteer could be of service during the 1918 pandemic, women's 'innate' abilities had to be imparted through specific training.

Operating in tandem with the assumption of women's universal ability to provide care, women were also called to the influenza front lines through an appeal to their putative sense of moral duty to their community. Women's natural sense of community duty was constructed through the language of ethical obligation, and through these calls women were interpellated into the role of caregiving subjects. One striking example of the use of moralistic language can be found in the *Courier*, which implored women to donate their time, declaring: 'If you have a soul, you will volunteer at once!' (*Courier* 1918c: 2). Thus, the decision to volunteer was not offered as an individual choice in which women could weigh the risks and benefits of volunteering given their own personal circumstances, but rather a social duty in which all 'good' women would unquestioningly offer their services for the benefit of the community. Indeed, the *Courier* took women's volunteerism for granted, noting: 'no doubt the response [to the call for volunteer nurses] will be in accordance with the need' (*Courier* 1918d: 4). This call left women at greater risk for influenza than their male counterparts.

While women were expected to put themselves at great personal risk for the community, there was little recognition of, or support for, the healthcare work performed by women. Newspaper reports acknowledged the efforts and skills of male doctors and politicians, claiming that their knowledge and expertise proved crucial in guiding the city in the face of chaos (*Courier* 1918e: 1). Yet the archival record shows that it was often highly trained, senior female nurses who were central to the management of emergency influenza services. In particular, Brantford's Medical Health Officer, Dr Pearson, appointed senior nurse Miss Kate McNeill as the supervisor of the temporary emergency hospital erected to handle the significant increase in patients (*The Expositor* 1918c: 1).

This emergency hospital, referred to as the Tabernacle, was the central site in Brantford for the treatment of those with the flu and, as such, often had over 150 patients at a time with only two or three trained nurses on staff (*The Expositor* 1918d: 6). As supervisor, McNeill had an extremely challenging situation to manage. Despite the importance of her position few articles specifically mentioned McNeill, or other women, when discussing the success of the healthcare services provided to the citizens of Brantford. For example, an article from *The Expositor* specifically draws attention to the work of men in the following statement about the civic ambulance services: '[we] should pay tribute not only to the efficiency, but the tenderness of the staff on the civic ambulance, remarkable work has been accomplished by these men during the present crisis' (*The Expositor* 1918a: 1). Yet the same article makes women's labour invisible in a statement about success at the hospital: 'the work at the Emergency hospital is being better organized, with a resultant increase of efficiency'. When women's efforts were acknowledged, these comments were often fleeting statements about nurses as a group such as 'nurses are taxed almost beyond human endurance' (*Courier* 1918f: 1). In comparison, most articles focused on the work and opinions of specific male civic leaders including the mayor, city councilors, members of the Board of Health and the Board of Trade, and medical men.

The impact of this particular construction of duty to care was that women in Brantford suffered higher levels of physical and emotional risk during the 1918 influenza pandemic. Newspaper articles in both local dailies consistently reported steady increases in the number of nurses, both trained and volunteer, who became ill during the most intense two-week period of the outbreak. For example, on 5 October 1918 it was reported in the *Courier* that two nurses were sick (*Courier* 1918g: 3); 11 days later reports stated there were at least 20 ill nurses, two of whom were head nurses at the emergency hospital (*Courier* 1918h: 1). In addition to the risk of becoming ill themselves, this arrangement placed a significant burden of risk on these women's families. Not only was the essential home-front labour of women missing during this time but nurses and volunteers were at risk of bringing illness home to other family members. The threat faced by women and their families when women took up nursing positions in the emergency hospital is particularly clear when this work is positioned in direct comparison to the advice provided to the citizens of Brantford:

> Avoid contact with other people so far as possible. Especially avoid crowds indoors
> . . . Avoid persons suffering from 'colds', sore throats and coughs . . . Sleep and work
> in clean, fresh air . . . Avoid visiting the sick (*The Expositor* 1918e: 5).

Brantford's experience of the 1918 influenza pandemic illustrates that the construction of duty to care as both moral and gendered meant that women were placed at greater personal risk during the pandemic. The duty to care remains a critical issue in contemporary pandemic planning and response. Although the notion of a duty to care may now be defined in narrower professional parameters, women still make up most front-line healthcare workers, and debates regarding the obligation of caregivers during pandemic situations remain ethical, rather than medical, in nature. Thus we argue that current stakeholders must reflect on these patterns in the historical record and question how moral and gendered constructions of the duty to care may operate to inscribe difference in contemporary pandemic planning and response.

Acknowledgements

This research was supported by the Canadian Program of Research on Ethics in a Pandemic, which was funded by the Canadian Institutes for Health Research (grant no. 457178), and the Lupina Foundation's Comparative Program on Health and Society. The authors wish to thank Annalise Clarkson for research assistance and the editors and reviewers for their suggestions.

Notes

1   Calculation based on statistics provided in Wisenthal (1983).
2   Jones (2008) comments that the scepticism towards volunteers may also have been used to bolster claims that nursing should be further professionalised.

References

Adams, T. (2010) Gender and feminization in healthcare professions, *Sociology Compass*, 4, 7, 454–65.
Courier (1918a) Churches, schools, theatres closed, 12 October.
Courier (1918b) Emergency hospital will provide for 100 influenza patients, 12 October.
Courier (1918c) Hospital board appeals for aid, 30 October.
Courier (1918d) Volunteer nurses, 15 October.
Courier (1918e) Mayor's advice to the public, 15 October.
Courier (1918f) Emergency hospital will provide for 100 influenza patients, 12 October.
Courier (1918g) No need for alarm, 5 October.
Courier (1918h) No improvement in flu situation, 16 October.
The Expositor (1918a) Volunteer workers are still needed at emergency hospital, 18 October.

The Expositor (1918b) First cycle of lessons in the emergency nursing complete, 21 October.

The Expositor (1918c) Dr Pearson, M.H.O., resigns, no abatement of epidemic, 15 October.

The Expositor (1918d) Demand for trained nurses is increasing, 21 October.

The Expositor (1918e) Precautions to be taken to avoid or ward off influenza, 15 October.

Joint Centre for Bioethics Pandemic Ethics Working Group (2008) The duty to care in a pandemic, *The American Journal of Bioethics*, 8, 8, 31–3.

Jones, E. (2008) *Influenza 1918: Disease, Death, and Struggle in Winnipeg*. Toronto: University of Toronto Press.

McPherson, K. (1996) *Bedside Matters: the Transformation of Canadian Nursing, 1900–1990*. Don Mills: Oxford University Press.

Ruderman, C., Tracy, C.S., Bensimon, C.M., Bernstein, M., *et al.* (2006) On pandemics and the duty to care: whose duty? who cares? *BMC Medical Ethics*, 7, 5, doi: 10.1186/1472-6939-7-5 (accessed 19 April 2012).

Wisenthal, M. (1983). Full-time teachers in public elementary and secondary schools, by sex, Canada and by province, selected years, 1867 to 1975 (Series W150–191). Statistics Canada website available at http://www5.statcan.gc.ca/bsolc/olc-cel/olc-cel?lang=eng&catno=11-516-X198300111318 (accessed 19 April 2012).

13

Flu frames

Karen Staniland and Greg Smith

Introduction

The H1N1 flu pandemic in the spring and summer of 2009 was a globally newsworthy story. In turn, the media attention given to the pandemic stimulated social scientific interest about its characterisation. According to health communication researchers, the manner in which the public was presented with information about pandemic flu was a key element in its management by nation-states and international health agencies. In many studies the investigation of the media characterisation was cast as a question about how it was 'framed'. This chapter investigates how the frame concept was used in these studies. In this way the authors hope to derive a better understanding of the sociological dimensions of news responses to the 2009 pandemic. The chapter concludes by reviewing some implications of the findings for models of moral panic (Cohen 1972/1973) and epidemic psychology (Strong 1990).

A brief history of a contested term

In sociology, Goffman's (1974) formulation remains classic. For Goffman (1974: 9) frames are 'schemata of interpretation' that individuals apply to address the question, 'What is *it* that's going on here?'[1] Is the activity being witnessed a joke, a deception, a misunderstanding, a greeting, a theatrical performance or what? Cognition, Goffman claims, owes more to such socially organised frames than is commonly thought. The way in which persons organise their activities is part of how they frame the world. Frames are 'organizational premises' that are 'sustained both in the mind and in activity' (Goffman 1974: 247).

As early as 1981, Goffman (1981: 67) dryly observed that plenty of researchers were using the frame concept with little mention of his writing on the subject. Goffman cited Tannen's (1979) survey, which showed that frame and cognate terms had become established in investigations carried out in anthropology, artificial intelligence, cognitive psychology, linguistics, social psychology and sociology. Often, there has been a tendency to conceptualise framing in more cognitive terms than Goffman proposed. Psychological ideas of 'script' and 'schema' stood at odds with the concentration on communicative conduct emphasised by Goffman. However, both psychological and sociological conceptions were underpinned by the idea that frames offer 'structures of expectations' (Tannen 1979) that

Pandemics and Emerging Infectious Diseases: The Sociological Agenda, First Edition. Edited by Robert Dingwall, Lily M. Hoffman and Karen Staniland. Chapters © 2013 The Authors. Book Compilation © 2013 Foundation for the Sociology of Health & Illness / John Wiley & Sons Ltd.

shape what we perceive in light of our prior experience and our acquaintance with how events and objects are organised. In psychology, the effect of frames on choices was demonstrated by Tversky and Kahneman's (1981) study where two equal scenarios, differently described as saving lives or causing deaths, attracted markedly different levels of support. Close affinities between Goffman's concept of frame and the concepts of 'schema' (Bartlett), 'habitus' (Bourdieu), 'perspective' (Shibutani) and 'thought style' (Fleck) were identified by Friedman (2011).

Of most direct relevance to this chapter is the work of media sociologists, who were quick to appreciate the utility of the notion for analysing how media texts are produced and understood. Tuchman (1978: 1) popularised the frame notion with her claim that 'News is a window on the world', noting that its content 'depends upon whether the window is large or small, has many panes or few, whether the glass is opaque or clear, whether the window faces a street or a backyard'. In one of the deftest definitions, Gitlin (1980: 6) suggested that frames were 'principles of selection, emphasis, and presentation composed of little tacit theories about what exists, what happens, and what matters'. This definition captured the textual dimension of framing. In everyday life, as Goffman noted, frames organise cognition and action. Media frames organise journalists' reports of the world and the understandings of those who rely on such reports. The critical task was to identify the frames that give order and pattern to news stories and to ask, why this frame and not another frame? Questions about how the news is framed have supplanted earlier concerns centring on the difficult notion of intentional bias (Schudson 2003: 35). The analytic terminology of frames allowed a less charged way of examining representations of pandemic flu.

The discipline with the strongest current claim to 'own' the frame concept is communication studies. Entman (1993) boldly claimed that communications was the field that could broker the fractured understandings of the framing concept created by its multidisciplinary uptake. This influential article (cited nearly 3500 times to date; Google Scholar, 7 May 2012) proposed that 'the concept of framing consistently offers a way to describe the power of the communicating text' (Entman 1993: 51). Underpinning framing are the notions of selection and salience. Frames select aspects of reality and make them more salient. For Entman (1993: 53) salience 'means making a piece of information more noticeable, meaningful or memorable to audiences'. Frames do at least four things: define problems, diagnose causes, make moral judgements and suggest remedies. They may be present in different places within the communication process: in communicators, texts, receivers and the culture (Entman 1993: 52).

In previous studies of news framing, two sets of conceptual distinctions have proved especially significant. The first, by Iyengar (1991), distinguished episodic and thematic frames to indicate the differing characteristics of news coverage. Episodic frames focused on the specifics of the occurrence reported: the when, where and how of the event. Thematic frames placed the occurrence in some wider context – the broader historical, social and economic background of the event. The second, by de Vreese (2005), distinguished issue-specific news frames (e.g. how the Intifada was framed, how an employment dispute was framed) from generic frames which were found recurrently across many issues and contexts, such as Iyengar's episodic/thematic distinction or Semetko and Valkenburg's (2000) five news frames ('conflict', 'human interest', 'attribution of responsibility', 'morality' and 'economic consequences'). These have proved valuable distinctions.

The attraction of the frame concept for those seeking to understand the news treatments of pandemic flu is clear. At moments of uncertainty and risk occasioned by the emergence of a new disease (Strong 1990), the frame concept pinpoints the 'little tacit theories about what exists, what happens, and what matters'. Following Gamson's (2001) suggestions (themselves echoing Hall's 1973/1980 encoding/decoding model and subsequent developments in the sociology of culture) we classified the studies in light of three aspects of frame analysis:

- Framing the flu: how did experts and media professionals build and reproduce news flu frames?
- Flu frames: what were the features of the frames through which the pandemic was represented in the news?
- Audiences and flu frames: how did audiences understand flu frames?

In seeking to determine how research studies used framing concepts to analyse media coverage of the 2009 pandemic, we initially conducted an electronic database and Google Scholar search for international published studies, using the search terms 'pandemic flu', 'swine flu', 'framing', 'H1N1' and 'media framing'. We selected a group of 15 studies published in 2010–2012. Table 1 summarises these in terms of (1) research problem, (2) sources of data and methods of analysis, and (3) framing conceptions employed. The criteria were that the studies addressed aspects of media representation and included a focus on, or relevance to, the concepts of frames and framing.

Framing the flu

Kenneth Burke noted the power of naming as a linguistic act: 'the mere act of naming an object or situation decrees that it is to be singled out as such-and-such rather than as something-other' (Burke 1941: 4). Vigso's (2010) article, 'Naming is framing', neatly puts this idea in sociological form. The contention is not new, however. In 1918 a *New York Times* editorial disputed the labelling of the flu pandemic as 'Spanish influenza' because it could not be proved that the disease was the same as the one that occurred many years earlier (Blakely 2003: 888). Vigso's (and Blakely's) point was that how the flu was initially framed stemmed from how it was named. The technical name, Influenza A (H1N1), was initially overshadowed by 'Mexican flu' and 'swine flu' in many countries. 'Naming controversies' were motivated by the interests of various national and international bodies in health and politics. The Mexican government rejected the name linking their country to the flu and sought to protect its trade and tourism interests by engaging in 'strategic reputation management'. The swine flu name played out in more complex ways – an Israeli government minister rejected the label because it meant that Jews would have to utter the name of an impure animal. The linking of a flu strain with pig keeping led China to place a ban on pork imports and to the Egyptian government ordering the slaughter of pigs (widely seen as form of harassment of Egypt's Christian minority who kept them). In the United States and across the European Union there was an immediate sensitivity to the threat to jobs and business interests. National and international agencies recognised that 'H1N1', difficult though it was to say, was preferable to the popular alternatives. Yet this proved hard to achieve. Vigso (2010) cites a study of Twitter messages in Sweden. Those originating from an official source of health information predominantly used H1N1 or a neutral variant; the messages from a national television station overwhelmingly used the value-laden descriptor 'swine flu'. Our own search of UK papers found that, for popular and 'broadsheet' newspapers alike, 'swine flu' was the most favoured descriptor, featuring in 2482 UK national newspaper headlines published between 27 April and 30 November 2009.

Table 1 *Framing the media representation of 2009 pandemic flu: summary of studies*

Reference, location of study	Research problem	Sources of data and methods of analysis	Framing conceptions employed
Chang (2010), United States	What frames did print journalists use to portray the 2009 H1N1 vaccine? How did vaccine supporters and opponents use frames in leading national newspapers?	Stories appearing in five influential US newspapers, April 2009–January 2010. Qualitative content analysis using the ATLAS. ti data storage software program. Examined word selection and content composition of news reporting to characterise media framing of the H1N1 vaccine	Problem frames: pro- and anti-vaccine frames (a total of 22 frames are identified)
Chew and Eysenbach (2010), global (but half of users are American)	Study aimed to '1) Monitor the use of the terms "H1N1" versus "swine flu" over time 2) conduct a content analysis of "tweets"; and 3) validate Twitter as a real-time content, sentiment, and public attention trend-tracking tool' (p. 1)	Content analysis of 2 million tweets during the 2009 H1N1 outbreak using manual coding and text-mining software	No explicit reference to framing concepts. Twitter content categories (see Chew and Eysenbach's table 1) could be translated into frame terms
Doudaki (2011), Greece and Cyprus	How did Greek and Cypriot newspapers represent the threat and actuality of pandemic flu?	Articles in the leading Greek and Cypriot newspapers. Content analysis principally, also discourse analysis and word searches	No explicit reference to framing concepts. Content categories: policy actors and actions; vaccination; schools and education (eight categories in total). Press acceptance of dominant frames of threats and risks
Fogarty et al. (2011), Australia	How did Australian television report H1N1 risk in 2009?	A content analysis of statements in Sydney television news items, April–October 2009	No explicit reference to framing concepts. News reports framed to reproduce public health sources

Study	Focus / Research question	Method	Framing findings
Hilton and Hunt (2011), UK	Examination of the content and 'framing' of the 2009 swine flu pandemic in UK newspapers	News stories and headlines in eight national newspapers. Quantitative manifest content analysis	Frame terminology marginal to analysis, although there is assessment of coverage as 'alarmist', 'reassuring' or 'neither'
Holland et al. (2012), Australia	Investigated the experiences of experts who were sources for the Australian news media during the pandemic	Qualitative semi-structured interviews with scientists and public health officials	Framing contests around different expert perceptions of risks of pandemic
Holland and Blood (2010), Australia	How was swine flu (and the actions and discussion it generated) reported in the Australian press?	Three significant Australian newspapers. Qualitative study of articles and their constituent elements	Uncertainty and risk, fear and danger, government preparedness, and beyond containment frames
Ibrahim, Normah, and Peng Kee (2010), Malaysia	What are the main frames used in newspaper reports of H1N1 in Malaysia? What differences exist between newspapers in the framing of the pandemic?	Content analysis of four Malaysian mainstream newspapers	Application of Semetko and Valkenburg's (2000) five generic frames: attribution of responsibility, conflict, human interest, economic consequences and morality
Lee and Basnyat (2012), Singapore	'To understand the use of press releases in news coverage of pandemics, this study traces the development of framing devices from a government public health agency's press releases to news stories about the 2009 H1N1 A influenza pandemic'	A content analysis of press releases from the Singapore Ministry of Health (MOH) matched to subsequent news articles about H1N1	Several 'framing devices': dominant frame, thematic versus episodic frames, emotion appeal, gain–loss frame, sourcing
Lopes et al. (2012), Portugal	A study of Influenza A stories and their sources in Portuguese newspapers during 2009	Content analysis of 655 articles in three national newspapers	No explicit reference to framing concepts. The study shows that the press accept dominant frames. Chaos abroad versus serenity and readiness at home

Table 1 *Continued*

Reference, location of study	*Research problem*	*Sources of data and methods of analysis*	*Framing conceptions employed*
Nerlich and Koteyko (2011), UK	Explores how the 2009 pandemic of swine flu (H1N1) intersected with issues of biosecurity in the context of an increasing entanglement between the spread of disease and the spread of information	Comparison of newspaper articles and blogs	Use of metaphors ('panic', 'crying wolf') and other metacommunicative framing devices
Oh *et al.* (2012), USA and Korea	Compares US and South Korean news coverage of the H1N1 pandemic to examine cross-cultural variations in attention cycle patterns, cited sources and news frames	A content analysis of H1N1 news coverage in three US and three Korean newspapers	Seven news frames; new evidence; attribution of responsibility; uncertainty; reassurance; consequence; bare statistics; action
Vigso (2010), Sweden	Why did the swine flu naming debate became so intense?	Discussion on the efforts at renaming the flu and explain it in a rhetorical and crisis communication context	Coombs' crisis management theory as well as framing theory and rhetoric
Wagner-Egger, *et al.* (2011), Switzerland	How did laypersons perceive the 'collectives' (i.e. groups, organisations, countries) implicated in the 2009 H1N1 outbreak?	Interviews with 47 Swiss adults in the early stages of the pandemic to elicit the risk posed by H1N1, its origins, consequences, protective measures, etc.	Dramaturgical framing of responses to identify heroes, victims and villains (Propp 1968)
Wang, Smith, and Worawongs (2010), worldwide	What frames figured in online news stories in the early stages of the H1N1 pandemic?	A total of 362 news stories sampled from Google News and coded. Descriptive statistics of sample characteristics	Five media frames: individual prevention, severity, transmission and stigmatising international students, stigmatising Mexicans, and infected region threat

The selection of an appropriate name for the flu highlights cultural sensitivities as well as the play of social, economic and political interests at work among a range of stakeholders. In Greece and Cyprus, newspapers stuck closely to World Health Organization (WHO) advice with fewer than 5% of articles using the name 'swine flu' (Doudaki 2011). However, in Malaysia 'swine flu' was frequently used in newspapers. It was felt that the dangers would be better understood if the Malay term for swine flu, *selsema babi*, was used (Ibrahim *et al.* 2010), hence *selsema babi* and Influenza A (H1N1) were used interchangeably. These contextual variations remind us that naming the flu was not a once-and-forever event but subject to processes of contestation. Changes over time were noted by Chew and Eysenbach's (2010) investigation of Twitter messages. Between 1 May and 31 December 2009, use of the WHO recommended term 'H1N1' increased from 8.8% to 40.5%. The precise scope of this finding is difficult to ascertain. While the 'Twittersphere' is in theory global, estimates suggest that the profile of users is younger, better educated and better-off than most nation-states' populations.

Naming is one manifest and initial dimension of the framing process. Other aspects of the production of news frames require investigation of the relationship of the published news item to its source. One way to address this is to observe or interview experts and media professionals. Only one study reviewed here took this approach. Holland *et al.* (2012) interviewed eight experts on infectious diseases who were frequently cited as sources for Australian newspapers and television in 2009. They found an element of dissension among the experts described as a 'framing contest', where a minority of experts interviewed felt that the others were 'toeing the party line', ignoring evidence that the pandemic was not as serious as government officials were convinced it was. Journalists commonly elicit differences among experts in order to make a 'balanced' story. In this case expert differences about the risks of swine flu did not become visible in news reports due to differential self-conceptions of the expert role and frustration with institutional constraints in playing the media game.

Another approach to the production of media frames is to consider the degree of concordance between the published news story and official press releases. Lopes *et al.* (2012) found heavy dependence by Portuguese journalists on the information provided by the national health ministry. Coverage overlooked other potential information sources, such as nurses, specialist Internet sites, blogs and citizens as patients, resulting in a 'huge spiral of silence' (Lopes *et al.* 2012: 23). Newspaper stories closely mirrored official sources because national health authorities, aware of the strategic importance of health communication, provided journalists with accessible packages of information that could readily be turned into news stories. Other studies (Holland and Blood 2010, Doudaki 2011, Duncan 2009) also indicated that, especially in the pandemic's early stages, there was extensive dependence on official sources of information and the frames they embodied.

A divergent picture of the framing process emerged in a Singapore study (Lee and Basnyat 2012) which found that journalists, faced with covering the uncertain risks of pandemic flu, saw themselves as agents and advocates of wider public health interests. Journalists actively filtered the information provided by their official sources. But in addition:

> the evolution from press release to news is marked by significant framing changes: expansion and diversification in dominant frames and emotion appeals, stronger thematic framing, more sources, conversion of loss into gain frames, and amplification of positive tone about the government's pandemic response efforts – suggesting that news stories are being framed to provide more than just 'the facts'. (Lee and Basnyat 2012: 11)

The heavy dependence on official sources suggests that national health authorities success-fully enacted WHO's (2004) Outbreak Communication Guidelines encouraging a strategy of early and active engagement with media organisations and staff. Yet the risk of journal-istic dependency on expert sources makes critical analysis of the information provided more difficult (but not, as the Singapore study showed, impossible).

The contribution of these studies to an understanding of how the flu was framed shows (1) naming varies according to cultural context, (2) lack of visibility of expert dissension in media reports, and (3) extensive dependence of news producers on official sources of infor-mation whose agenda could be simply reproduced (as in Portugal and Greece) or proactively expanded (Singapore) by the press.

Flu frames

The notion of the 'problem frame' suggests that news media operate with discourses assum-ing that 'danger and risk are a central feature of the effective environment' (Altheide 1997: 648). Chang's (2010) analysis of H1N1 pro- and anti-vaccination problem frames in five leading US newspapers' coverage identified 22 different frames used by advocates and opponents of vaccination. Tracking their shifting prominence in a nine-month period begin-ning April 2009, Chang found that pro-vaccine frames stressed protective factors while anti-vaccine frames expressed safety concerns. The greater prevalence and consistency of provaccine frames across the period of the study led to these frames becoming dominant in newspaper coverage. However, the continuing prominence of the low availability of vaccine frame may have diluted the efforts of public health officials to get across their message that the vaccine would save lives.

Problem frames were not the only frames figuring in responses to pandemic flu. They were sometimes complemented by frames that emphasised government preparedness to deal appropriately with any of the risks confronting the nation, whether pandemic flu, terrorism or disaster (Stephenson and Jamieson 2009). In Portugal, especially at the start of the out-break, newspapers adopted a dual framing, presenting an 'alarming scenario' abroad while emphasising the 'serenity' and readiness of the Portuguese authorities' response at home (Lopes *et al.* 2012: 24). This pattern was found elsewhere. Holland and Blood (2010) acknowledge the presence of risk and fear frames in initial Australian press coverage but suggest that the frames that quickly became dominant were 'government preparedness' and 'beyond containment'. In advance of the arrival of the virus, stories emphasised the plans that were in place to deal with the health crisis. Once cases started to appear in Australia, a 'beyond containment' frame became dominant. Press stories, to some extent mirroring WHO's own prediction, portrayed a rampant virus spreading at a rate that officials could not control. Reassuring stories ('just another flu') were subordinated to those that played up the public's fears ('experts warn of mutation').

Hilton and Hunt (2011) acknowledged the media's important role as a disseminator of scientific information about risk perception. They noted that 'perspectives or 'frames' influ-ence what are included or excluded from stories and can misrepresent the scientific evi-dence'. For example, in October 2009, when swine flu cases peaked a second time, newspaper interest decreased. The rating of articles and headlines separately as 'alarmist', 'reassuring' or 'neither' shows consistently high scores for 'neither' across the 12-month period of the study. Thus, Hilton and Hunt conclude that in the UK there was little media 'over-hyping' of the swine flu pandemic. Reporting was largely measured and responsible.

Two studies of newspaper representations of the pandemic in South East Asia drew upon established frame analytic terminology. Ibrahim *et al.* (2010) adopted Semetko and

Valkenburg's (2000) generic news frames in order to ascertain how they were configured in the context of Malaysian newspaper coverage of the pandemic. Here, the responsibility frame scored highest, followed by the morality, human interest, conflict and economic consequences frames. In short, they found that all the newspapers wanted the government to take responsibility for solving the problems associated with the pandemic. Conversely, the economic consequences of the pandemic did not receive much attention in Malaysian news stories. Concerns with moral prescriptions, human interest and conflict between individuals, groups and institutions attracted moderate scores. Lee and Basnyat (2012) used Iyengar's (1991) distinction between episodic and thematic framing as one of their six coding categories. They found that journalists increased the proportion of thematic framing in their stories – they provided more context and background to the issues around the pandemic than was present in Ministry of Health press releases. Like Ibrahim *et al.* (2010), this study's use of established frame terms encourages comparisons between health communication news and other types of news.

The majority of studies examined representations in the print press. However, the increasing role of the internet as a favoured source of health information was acknowledged. Chew and Eysenbach (2010) presented a method for tracing collective sentiments and misinformation about the pandemic presented on Twitter but was not itself directly concerned with news reporting. Wang *et al.* (2010) investigated media frames in the reporting found in Google News, in the early stage of the pandemic between March and June 2009. The most frequent of the five frames identified in online news stories (Table 1) was the 'transmission' and 'stigmatising international students' frame. These two frames showed the greatest stability across the sample period. The latter frame indicated that international students continued to be stigmatised even when people came to know more about the sources of the disease. The 'individual prevention', 'severity' and 'infected region' frames, on the other hand, were more prominent in stories in the earliest part of the sample period.

Oh *et al.* (2012) is the only study in the sample with an explicit comparative dimension. Of the seven frames (Table 1) figuring in their analysis of the pandemic, the 'attribution of responsibility' frame was most frequent in the US press reporting, while the 'bare statistics' frame was most prominent in Korean coverage. This finding underlined the contrast in cultural belief between the activist United States, where the belief was that the government had a responsibility to fight the epidemic, and Korea, where fatalistic views were more commonplace and thus news reporting concentrated on changes in the statistics charting the course of the pandemic.

Fogarty *et al.* (2011) examined Australian television coverage. Despite swine flu's uncertain trajectory and television's production culture that notoriously prizes 'seven-second soundbites' and simple, readily understandable information, reporting was found to be reassuring and non-alarmist. The study identified that the majority of reports were made by broadcast journalists, government representatives such as medical officers, and public health and infectious disease experts. Media reporting frames in this context consisted of 'updates and developments, mainly focussed on case increases' (Fogarty *et al.* 2011: 187). Television's framing of pandemic flu, at least in Australia, seemed more measured and less sensational than its press counterpart.

While the studies reviewed indicate widespread recognition of the importance of frames and framing for understanding the news, systematic application of existing theoretical knowledge about news frames across this collection of studies was uneven. Several studies (Ibrahim *et al.* 2010, Lee and Basnyat 2012, Oh *et al.* 2012, Wang *et al.* 2010) used or adapted existing conceptual distinctions. In some others (e.g. Chew and Eysenbach 2010, Fogarty *et al.* 2011, Hilton and Hunt 2011, Lopes *et al.* 2012) framing terminology was either marginal or could readily have been applied to strengthen the analysis presented. Further use of framing analysis would have enhanced the opportunities for comparison with other types of crisis news (cf. An and Gower 2009). Such comparative and generalising ambitions depend to a degree on deductive theorising (testing out existing frames) and are in tension with the aim of inductively deriving frames in order to illuminate the particularities of pandemic framing in specific contexts (e.g. the approaches taken by Chang 2010, Holland and Blood 2010, and Wang *et al.* 2010 that were aimed at discovering new frames appropriate to their topic-matter). Of course, part of the attraction of the frame concept is its flexibility (Reese 2001) and tractability to a variety of explanatory endeavours. Perri 6 (2005) has argued that framing analyses are descriptive and not properly explanatory until they are anchored into some theoretical context (neo-Durkheimian institutional theory for Perri 6, attention cycles for Oh *et al.* 2012).

Our sample of studies tends to take the entire news article as the unit of analysis. The varying significance of the constituent elements of articles was not always recognised by this approach. However, Doudaki (2011) attended to the front page placement of articles; Hilton and Hunt (2011) separately coded the headlines and the main body of reports; and Holland and Blood (2010) adopted an open-ended qualitative approach attentive to the framing power of headlines, lead paragraphs, and quoted sources of information and opinion. Visual material was largely ignored. In our own investigation of 80 UK national newspaper front page stories, only 19 images were found, manifesting a limited visual repertoire. The most common image was a surgically masked face.

Audiences and flu frames

Many framing studies seem premised on the notion that the encoded news frame is so compelling that audiences can only make a single sense of it. A contrasting view, derived from the encoding/decoding tradition of British cultural studies, contends that frames are a 'structured polysemy' – they can be read in various ways but these are 'structured in dominance'. There are both 'preferred readings' and negotiated or oppositional readings that may be made by members of different social groupings (Hall [1973], 1980/1980). The sense that readers make of news frames cannot be simply assumed but becomes a matter of empirical examination.

If the chief source of information to laypersons about the pandemic is the mass media, how can media impact on laypersons' framing of H1N1 be specified? Wagner-Egger *et al.*'s (2011) interviews with French-speaking Swiss citizens in May–June 2009 identified key categories of collectivity. The 'heroes' of the unfolding drama were the experts, especially the researchers and the physicians who charted its course, prepared a vaccination and gave practical advice. The 'villains' were the media who stoked up people's fears and the big corporations, notably the pharmaceutical industry, which profited from the pandemic. The 'victims' were the poorer countries that lacked the resources to cope properly with their people's needs. Victims, however, were seen ambivalently. They were held culpable because of their lack of hygiene, discipline or 'culture'. This dramaturgical framing of heroes, villains and victims was:

> at odds with the scientific way of framing disease threat, i.e. as an abstract risk. At least some of the misunderstandings of science attributed to laypersons may be due to these potentially incommensurable frames, rather than to deficits in understanding. (Wagner-Egger *et al.* 2010: 474–5)

The contested reception and interpretation of flu news frames was addressed by Nerlich and Koteyko's (2011) study of the UK swine flu outbreak. They emphasised the unique context of the 2009 outbreak. First, there were the repeated warnings of avian-type flu pandemic from 2004 onwards that did not materialise and encouraged scepticism towards claims about the risks of swine flu when it first appeared. Second, the use of digital technologies, especially social media such as Twitter and blogging, interacted with traditional news sources in the press and television in the UK. Media commentary, especially in the early stages of the pandemic, focused not only on the nature of the flu threat ('biosecurity concerns'), but also on how perception of these threats was changed by the impact of social media, an impact that was itself a topic of mass and social media discussion ('metacommunication').

Biosecurity concerns were reflected in UK media coverage during April and May 2009, which repeated the pattern of previous outbreaks of infectious diseases. Initially alarmist reporting about the risks was followed by more measured and moderate accounts. What was new was the rise of metacommunicative reporting in which journalists and bloggers self-referentially reflected upon the role of their own reporting on the creation of the threats and risks posed by the pandemic. Print media discourses first blamed the officials (principally at WHO), then blamed the media ('scaremongering', 'crying wolf'), then shifted to a recognition of how 'we are hooked on hype' and ever willing to find new sources of panic. Meanwhile, the blogosphere identified the hype potential of pandemic flu weeks before the print media did. The discourses of both print and blogs concentrated on the dangers of 'panic fatigue' kicking in at just the point where actual flu cases transformed speculative risks into real ones. Nerlich and Koteyko show the complex interactions between social media and print journalism as both parties, in a situation of uncertainty about the flu's trajectory, attempted to decode dominant frames and offered a range of 'negotiated' or 'oppositional' framings. In a globalised world of mobilities and flows, where established boundaries become porous, it seems that new disease threats move rapidly from place to place.

There are at least two areas of audience-oriented research into pandemic frames warranting further inquiry. One is to take some of the judgements made by coders of news reports and make them an issue for exploration by the readers of these reports (e.g. via interviews or focus groups). Several papers referred to versions of Ungar's (2008) distinction between alarming and reassuring discourses or frames. For example, Hilton and Hunt (2011) use this distinction in order to discover that over three-quarters of UK coverage is 'neither', thus concluding that swine flu was not over-hyped. But from Goffman we might learn that an alarming/reassuring judgement is not simply a property of a text: it arises from the interaction of a reader and a text. Soliciting people's views is just as necessary as textual analysis. Second, text-based frame analyses need to take account of the various ways in which people read newspapers. Readers do not systematically read news articles from beginning to end. As readers pick up a newspaper and scan its contents, their attention is caught first by headlines and pictures. Singly and in conjunction, they direct the reader to newspaper stories of potential interest. Headlines and pictures are a potent source of first impressions that can play a significant role in shaping readers' attitudes towards the story's topic.

Conclusion: Frames, moral panics, and epidemic psychologies

Since most of the articles reviewed were conducted under the auspices of communication studies, the conjecture was that they would provide strong analyses of the content of frames but would be less convincing on the more sociological territory of production and consumption of texts. This proved to be only partially true. While questions of frame production on the one hand, and the interpretation and challenging of frames on the other hand, were not at the forefront of many analyses, they were not neglected.

Sociologists cannot help but notice the raised social anxieties provoked by the onset of an epidemic. When those anxieties are presented through colourful and exaggerated press reports, sociologists typically suspect the presence of media amplification and moral panic (Cohen [1972], 1973/1973). Moral panic theory helps to specify a sociological interest in epidemics as matters of representation. However, the major difficulty with straightforwardly applying the theory is the difficulty in identifying a single, epidemic-specific folk devil around which the moral panic can be mobilised. It is possible to identify 'heroes, villains and victims' (Wagner-Egger *et al.* 2011) that indicate the pervasive moralisation of the perception of swine flu. The occupants of these categories vary over time and place (big pharma for the Swiss; Mexicans and travellers for Americans). Also, in the case of emerging infectious diseases such as H1N1, there was not the scope for exaggerated claims, since, in the face of uncertainty, the wide support for medical expertise provides the default. Nevertheless, moral panic theory draws attention to the ways in which mediatised representations help to shape the public's conception of the nature of problems such as epidemics. Sociological interest is thus directed towards the characteristics of response to epidemics, not simply as threats to people's health or to the economy, but to the social order itself.

This is the point of departure for Strong's (1990) model of 'epidemic psychology'. Strong identified elements of the 'distinctive collective psychology' that accompanied outbreaks of epidemic diseases. He proposed three psycho-social epidemics that run alongside the embodied kinds: an epidemic of fear, suspicion and stigmatisation; an epidemic of interpretation, explanation and moralisation; and an epidemic of proposals and action. Just as all members of a society are vulnerable to an epidemic in their midst, so too are all members of society vulnerable to the fears and open to the explanations and calls for action that an epidemic unleashes. Based on studies of medieval plagues and the AIDS scares of the 1980s, Strong's model was designed to identify the kinds of responses that might accompany any particular outbreak of an epidemic. It offered an ideal type of what occurs in the wild when the scope and risks of a novel disease are not yet determined. As we indicated, the initially alarmist print news frames did occur in several countries. Much national and international planning was premised on the possibility of an apocalyptic event of 1918 proportions. The short-lived alarmist framing is in accord with Strong's epidemic of fear. As our discussion of framing the flu demonstrated, health authorities sought to control the epidemics of fear and explanation through their association with medical expertise and their monopoly control of remedial actions to combat spread of the disease. When framing contests emerged, around vaccination or expert opinion, the home side won. The metacommunicative (Nerlich and Koteyko 2011) framing of the media's role in the epidemic of fear as a 'media pandemic' has interesting implications for Strong's model. The new media technologies compress Strong's three psycho-social epidemics, reducing their temporal phasing and complicating the communicative processes between the public, the media and experts. These are some of the ways that the study of flu frames presents an alternative and interesting way to uncover the specific forms of epidemic psychologies in different social and cultural contexts.

Acknowledgements

The authors would like to thank Professor Robert Dingwall and the anonymous reviewers for comments on an earlier draft of this chapter.

Note

1 Goffman (1974: 9) italicises 'it' in recognition of how the question, as stated, assumes a single answer. Goffman (1974: 21) also acknowledges that more than one frame may be operating simultaneously.

References

Altheide, D.L. (1997) The news media, the problem frame and the production of fear, *Sociological Quarterly*, 38, 4, 647–68.

An, S. and Gower, K. (2009) How do the news media frame crises? A content analysis of crisis news coverage, *Public Relations Review*, 35, 107–12.

Blakely, D. (2003) Social construction of three influenza pandemics in the New York Times, *Journalism and Mass Communication Quarterly*, 80, 884–902.

Burke, K. (1941) *The Philosophy of Literary Form: Studies in Symbolic Action*. Baton Rouge, LA: Louisiana State.

Chang, J. (2010) *How U.S. Newspapers Frame the 2009 H1N1 Vaccine*. http://nature.berkeley.edu/classes/es196/projects/2010final/ChangJ_2010.pdf/.

Chew, C. and Eysenbach, G. (2010) Pandemics in the age of Twitter: content analysis of tweets during the 2009 H1N1 outbreak, *PLoS ONE*, 5, 11, e14118.

Cohen, S. ([1972] 1973) *Folk Devils and Moral Panics [1972]*. London: Paladin.

De Vreese, C.H. (2005) News framing: theory and typology, *Information Design Journal and Document Design*, 13, 1, 51–62.

Doudaki, V. (2011) Representations of disease and threat: the case of swine flu in Greece and in Cyprus. In Baxter, L. and Braescu, P. (eds) *Fear Within Melting Boundaries*. Oxford: Inter-Disciplinary Press.

Duncan, B. (2009) How the media reported the first days of the pandemic: (H1N1) 2009: results of a EU wide media analysis, *Eurosurveillance*, 14, 30, 1–3.

Entman, R.M. (1993) Framing: toward clarification of a fractured paradigm, *Journal of Communication*, 43, 4, 51–8.

Fogarty, A.S., Holland, K., Imison, M.R., Blood, R., Chapman, S. and Holding, S. (2011) Communicating uncertainty – how Australian television reported H1N1 risk in 2009: a content analysis, *BMC Public Health*. http://www.ncbi.nlm.nih.gov/pmc/articles/PMC3079644/.

Friedman, A. (2011) Toward a sociology of perception: sight, sex, and gender, *Cultural Sociology*, 5, 187–206.

Gamson, W. (2001) Foreword. In Reese, S.D. *et al.* (eds) *Framing Public Life: Perspectives on Media and Our Understanding of the Social World*. London: Taylor & Francis.

Gitlin, T. (1980) *The Whole World is Watching*. Berkeley, CA: University of California Press.

Goffman, E. (1974) *Frame Analysis: An Essay on the Organization of Experience*. New York, NY: Harper.

Goffman, E. (1981) A reply to Denzin and Keller, *Contemporary Sociology*, 10, 1, 60–8.

Hall, S. ([1973] 1980) Encoding/decoding. In Hall, S., Hobson, D., Lowe, A. and Willis, P. (eds) *Culture, Media, Language: Working Papers in Cultural Studies*, 1972–79. London: Hutchinson.

Hilton, S. and Hunt, K. (2011) UK newspapers' representations of the 2009–10 outbreak of swine flu: one health scare not over-hyped by the media?, *Journal of Epidemiological Community Health*, 65, 941–6.

Holland, K. and Blood, R.W. (2010) Not just another flu? The framing of swine flu in the Australian Press. In McCallum, K. (ed.) *Media, Democracy and Change*. Proceedings of the Australian and New Zealand Communications Association Annual Conference, Canberra, ACT, Australia, 7–9 July 2010. http://www.anzca.net/conferences/anzca10-conference.html/.

Holland, K., Blood, R., Imison, M., Chapman, S. and Fogarty, A. (2012) Risk, expert uncertainty, and Australian news media: public and private faces of expert opinion during the 2009 swine flu pandemic, *Journal of Risk Research*, 15, 6, 1–15.

Ibrahim, F., Normah, M. and Peng Kee, C. (2010) Framing a pandemic: analysis of Malaysian mainstream newspapers in the H1N1 coverage. Paper presented at the International Communication Association 2010 Preconference – Health Communication Campaigns: Issues and Strategies in Asia, Australia and Southeast Asia, 22 June 2010. Singapore: Singapore Health Promotion Board.

Iyengar, S. (1991) *Is Anyone Responsible? How Television Frames Political Issues*. Chicago, IL: University of Chicago Press.

Lee, S. and Basnyat, I. (2012) From press release to news: mapping the framing of the 2009 H1N1 A influenza pandemic, *Health Communication*, doi:10.1080/10410236.2012.658550. http://dx.doi.org/1 0.1080/10410236.2012.658550/.

Lopes, F., Ruão, T., Marinho, S. and Araújo, R. (2012) Media pandemic: Influenza A in Portuguese newspapers, *International Journal of Healthcare Management*, 5, 1, 19–27.

Nerlich, B. and Koteyko, N. (2011) Crying wolf? Biosecurity and metacommunication in the context of the 2009 swine flu pandemic, *Health and Place*, 18, 4, 710–7.

Oh, H.J., Hove, T., Paek, H.J., Lee, B., Lee, H. and Song, S.K. (2012) Attention cycles and the H1N1 pandemic: a cross-national study of US and Korean newspaper coverage, *Asian Journal of Communication*, 22, 2, 214–32.

Perri 6 (2005) What's in a frame? Social organization, risk perception and the sociology of knowledge, *Journal of Risk Research*, 8, 2, 91–118.

Propp, V. (1968) *The Morphology of the Folk Tale [originally published in Russian, 1928]*. Austin: University of Texas Press.

Reese, S. (2001) Prologue – Framing public life: a bridging model for media research. In Reese, S., Gandy, O. and Grant, A. (eds) *Framing Public Life: Perspectives on Media and Our Understanding of the Social World*. Mahwah, NJ: Lawrence Erlbaum.

Schudson, M. (2003) *The Sociology of News*. New York, NY: Norton.

Semetko, H. and Valkenburg, P. (2000) Framing European politics: a content analysis of press and television news, *Journal of Communication*, 50, 2, 93–109.

Stephenson, N. and Jamieson, M. (2009) Securitising health: Australian newspaper coverage of pandemic influenza, *Sociology of Health & Illness*, 31, 4, 525–39.

Strong, P. (1990) Epidemic psychology: a model, *Sociology of Health & Illness*, 12, 249–59.

Tannen, D. (1979) What's in a frame? Surface evidence for underlying expectations. In Freedle, R. (ed.) *New Directions in Discourse Processing*. Norwood, NJ: Ablex.

Tuchman, G. (1978) *Making News: A Study in the Construction of Reality*. New York, NY: Free Press.

Tversky, A. and Kahneman, D. (1981) The framing of decisions and the psychology of choice, *Science, n.s.*, 211, 4481, 453–8.

Ungar, S. (2008) Global bird flu communication: hot crisis and media reassurance, *Science Communication*, 29, 4, 472–97.

Vigso, O. (2010) Naming is framing: swine flu, new flu, and A (H1N1), *Observatorio (OBS*) Journal*, 4, 3, 229–41.

Wagner-Egger, P., Bangerter, A., Gilles, I., Green, E., Rigaud, D., Krings, F., Staerklé, C. and Clémence, A. (2011) Lay perceptions of collectives at the outbreak of the H1N1 epidemic: heroes, villains and victims, *Public Understanding of Science*, 20, 461–76.

Wang, W., Smith, R. and Worawongs, W. (2010) Googling the H1N1 flu: investigating media frames in online news coverage of the flu pandemic. Paper presented at the Annual Meeting of the International Communication Association, Suntec City, Singapore, 22 June 2010. http://www.allacademic.com/meta/p405189_index.html/.

World Health Organization (WHO) (2004) *Best Practices for Communicating with the Public During an Outbreak*. Report of the WHO Expert Consultation on Outbreak Communications, Singapore, 21–23 September 2004.

14

Attention to the media and worry over becoming infected: the case of the Swine Flu (H1N1) Epidemic of 2009

Gustavo S. Mesch, Kent P. Schwirian and Tanya Kolobov

Introduction

In the United States in 2009 there was a major outbreak of H1N1 (Swine Flu). By the end of the year more than 61 million were affected by the virus, 275,000 were hospitalised and 12,500 had died. Whenever a pandemic strikes, a wave of mass media reports spread the story, often in the most overstated and alarming tones (Bomlitz and Brezis 2008). As news of the contagion is disseminated, fear or worry over infection often breaks out in segments of the population (Alcabes 2009). Fear of infection may help individuals define the personal significance of the event and influence their decisions to seek protective immunisation (Altheide and Michalowski 1999, Setbon and Raude 2010).

In this chapter we focus on the H1N1 outbreak of 2009; our concern is with the link between attention to the media and fear. Our research question is, with social category membership controlled, to what extent did attention to media reports about the H1N1 outbreak contribute to a sense of worry or concern over the possibility of infection?

While the initial effect of exposure to media over-reporting is well known in the literature on cultivation effects, less is known about the long term association of media reporting to public concern (Shrum 2007). It is possible that after the public gathers knowledge from the media, public interest in the news decreases. If it decreases, does worry remain associated with media or are other factors better explanations of public concern?

Theory, hypothesis and methods

Two theoretical models inform our research – the media agenda-setting theory (Dearing and Rogers 1996), and the health belief model (Rosenstock 1960, Becker 1974). The media agenda-setting perspective argues that the attention and salience given to an issue in media coverage has an effect on which issues people pay attention to and on which they think is important. The health belief model argues that media reports are among the cues to action that shape what people perceive as a health threat. Furthermore, the model argues that the perception may differ by social categories. On the basis of these two models we hypothesise, controlling for the effects of social category membership, that those who followed H1N1 closely in the media were more interested in it and were more likely to be worried about

Pandemics and Emerging Infectious Diseases: The Sociological Agenda, First Edition. Edited by Robert Dingwall, Lily M. Hoffman and Karen Staniland. Chapters © 2013 The Authors. Book Compilation © 2013 Foundation for the Sociology of Health & Illness / John Wiley & Sons Ltd.

the possibility of becoming infected. Furthermore, media agenda setting theory argues that issue reporting decreases over time. Given this reduction in media attention, we hypothesise that net of the effect of social category membership following the media and being interested in H1N1 will have a lesser effect on worry at a later stage.

Our survey data are from two independent random digit dial samples representative of the US population (News Interest Index Survey) conducted by the Pew Research Center for People & the Press (http://people press.org/methodology/sampling). The samples included identical questions on the respondent's concern about infection with H1N1 and interest in the news about it. The first sampling took place from 1 May to 4 May 2009 (N = 1004). This was the time at which the spring H1N1 outbreak was slackening and the news coverage of it had initially peaked. The second sampling was conducted from 28 August to 31 August 2009 (N = 1006). This was the period in which both flu activity and media coverage began to increase after the summer lull (Mesch *et al.* 2011). Between the two samplings the World Health Organization (WHO) raised the pandemic alert for the outbreak from phase 5 to 6.

The dependent variable was 'Worried in the possibility of exposure to swine flu' (Worried). In the survey respondents were asked: 'How worried are you that you or someone in your family will be exposed to this flu – very worried, somewhat worried, not too worried, or not worried at all?' The scale was from 1 = 'Very worried' to 4 = 'Not worried at all'. Because of the skewed distribution of responses we converted it to a dummy variable with: 1 = 'Worried', 0 = 'Not worried'. Fear may be expressed for both oneself and generalised for others, such as family members. Often fear for significant others is higher than fear for oneself, therefore we used a measure that informs on worry of exposure that includes both self and others (War and Ellison 2000).

Two independent variables were used to investigate the perceived effect of exposure to the media on the perceived concern of infection. As H1N1 flu was declared a global pandemic condition by the WHO, we used measures indicating following the news on both local and global prevalence. The first was 'Interest in information about H1N1' (Interest). The respondents were asked to indicate if they happened to follow the outbreak of swine flu in different parts of the world very closely, fairly closely, not too closely, or not at all closely?

Because of the skewed distribution of the responses a dummy variable was created and coded 1 = 'Interested', 0 = 'Not interested'.

The second independent variable was the comparative extent of 'following information about swine flu' (Followed). The respondents were asked to 'indicate which one of the stories I just mentioned have you followed most closely, or is there another story you've been following more closely?' One of the possibilities was: 'The outbreak of swine flu in different parts of the world'. For responses to this question we created a new variable with 1 = 'Follow the swine flu', 0 = 'Not follow the swine flu'.

As additional modifying variables we used: race, gender, age, family status, education, number of children aged under 18, and income and family size (See Table 2 for categories).

Findings

Table 1 presents the percentage of respondents at each time who were worried about infection from H1N1 and the two measures of interest in the news about H1N1. The results indicate that the percentage of worried individuals increased during the period from 35.9

Table 1 *Worry and media*

	May 2009 (%)	August 2009 (%)
Worried	35.9	44.8
Follow closely Swine Flu news vs. other news	39.1	10.3
(Interest) From all stories most interested in Swine Flu stories	43.1	26.4

to 44.8 per cent as would normally be expected with the accumulation of media reports over the period. Yet the percentage of individuals that followed the H1N1 news more closely than other stories decreased from 39.1 to 10.3 per cent. Furthermore, the percentage of individuals replying that the reports they followed most closely were on H1N1 also decreased from 43.1 per cent of the sample to 26.4 per cent. These differences were all statistically significant and suggest that: (1) as the disease outbreak continued, there was an increasing percentage of people expressing concern over becoming exposed; and (2) once interest in and worry about H1N1 were established in media consumers, additional stories about H1N1 became simply further variations on the same theme and somewhat less interesting than other topics.

Table 2 shows that most social categories of people were becoming increasingly worried between May and August. The extent of worry was highest among females, those over 65 years, and those whose families were large – those with six or more children. Worry declined only among Black and Hispanic respondents, but even for them the percentage worried remained comparatively high. Table 2 also shows that those who followed and had interest in H1N1 remained markedly worried about it while those who were neither interested in H1N1 news or followed it actually became increasingly worried. On the basis of the results shown in Tables 1 and 2, we suggest a possible two-step process of concern – one that spreads throughout the population at the outbreak led by media reporting, and one later on as media interest decreases, but as a general social contextual effect in which social networks and personal experience become important.

In testing our hypotheses (see Table 3) our analytic strategy had two steps. For each of the two surveys (May 2009 and August 2009) we conducted two multivariate analyses predicting the likelihood that the respondents expressed worry that they or someone in their family would be exposed to swine flu (H1N1). In the first model we used the independent variable measuring the extent to which the respondent followed H1N1. The second model used the degree of interest in H1N1. The two variables have only a low correlation with each other. By introducing the independent variables separately in the two equations, each model represents an independent test of the hypothesis. There is no significant interaction effect of the two when they are in the same equation (not shown).

The results for May 2009 in Table 3 show that within each model with the social category measures controlled, the independent variable had a significant relationship with worry of exposure. In model 1 the odds ratio for 'Followed' was 1.93 ($p < 0.01$) and in Model 2 the odds ratio for 'Interest' is 3.36 ($p < 0.01$). In addition, with 'Followed' and 'Interest' controlled several of the social category variables were associated with worry. In the May survey only, there were measures of exposure to print, electronic and digital media. The results indicated that exposure to cable TV news increased the likelihood of concern with infection as compared to exposure to print and digital media. The introduction of media variables did not change the effect of the independent measures (analysis not shown).

Table 2 *Concern with becoming sick (worried) by social category*

Variables	May 2009 (%)	August 2009 (%)	Z
Gender			
Male	31.2	34.9%	−1.76
Female	40.6	54.1%	−6.06**
Age			
18–29	32.5	36.1	−1.70
30–49	36.3	44.0	−3.52**
50–64	39.8	48.5	−3.93**
65+	32.5	52.2	−8.94**
Family status			
Married	34.2	43.7	−4.37**
Not married	38.6	46.8	−3.72**
Education			
College graduate	35.8	41.0	−2.40**
Some college	33.2	44.9	−5.38**
High school or less	37.6	49.6	−5.42**
Family size			
1–2	33.0	46.6	−6.23**
3–5	39.3	42.0	−1.23
6+	25.0	53.7	−13.17**
Have children 0–6			
Yes	36.1	49.3	−5.98**
No	34.8%	43.7	−4.09**
Have children 6–11			
Yes	35.5	47.3	−5.37**
No	35.2	44.0	−4.03**
Have children 11–17			
Yes	32.1	46.3	−6.52**
No	35.9	44.5	−3.93**
Income			
Less than $30,000	35.2	46.1	−4.97**
$30,000–$49,999	40.6	47.1	−2.94**
$50,000–$74,000	30.4	43.6	−6.13**
$75,000+	32.9	42.0	−4.21**
Race			
White	30.6	46.3	−7.23**
Black	54.5	48.8	2.56**
Asian	47.4	−	
Hispanic	42.9	38.2	2.15*
Followed Swine flu			
Yes	42.7	44.6	−0.86
No	31.7	44.9	−6.09**
Interest Swine Flu			
Yes	49.30	64.20	−6.74**
No	26.00	37.80	−5.67**

*p < 0.05, **p < 0.01.

Table 3 *Logistic regressions predicting concern with becoming sick (worried)*

| | May 2009 | | | | | | August 2009 | | | | | |
| | Model 1 | | | Model 2 | | | Model 1 | | | Model 2 | | |
	B	S.E.	Odds	B	S.E.	Odds	B	S.E.	Odds	B	S.E.	Odds
Age	0.07	0.03	1.08*	0.03	0.03	1.03	0.13	0.03	1.14**	0.12	0.03	1.13**
male	-0.73	0.18	0.48**	-0.78	0.18	0.46**	-0.71	0.16	0.48**	-0.71	0.16	0.48**
married	-0.51	0.23	0.59*	-0.45	0.24	0.63*	-0.46	0.20	0.62*	-0.45	0.16	0.48**
Some college[1]	-0.33	0.24	0.71	-0.33	0.25	0.71	-0.36	0.21	0.69	-0.29	0.21	0.74
Graduate	-0.16	0.23	0.86	-0.02	0.23	0.97	-0.20	0.21	0.81	-0.26	0.21	0.76
Family size	0.18	0.09	1.19*	0.16	0.09	1.17*	0.11	0.07	1.12	0.14	0.08	1.15
Children 6–11[2]	-0.37	0.24	0.68	-0.36	0.25	0.69	0.16	0.21	1.17	0.15	0.22	1.16
Children 11–17	-0.75	0.25	0.46**	-0.80	0.25	0.44**	0.008	0.20	1.008	-0.01	0.21	0.98
Less than average income[3]	.081	0.28	2.26**	0.82	0.29	2.29**	0.10	0.25	1.11	0.21	0.26	1.24
Average income	0.29	0.30	1.34	0.20	0.31	1.22	-0.16	0.26	0.85	-0.07	0.27	0.92
High income	0.69	0.29	2.002*	0.51	0.29	1.66	-0.03	0.25	0.96	0.02	0.26	1.13
Black[4]	1.39	0.28	4.01**	1.25	0.28	3.48**	0.23	0.25	1.26	-0.02	0.18	0.01
Asian	0.87	0.62	2.38	0.52	0.63	1.68	1.13	1.86	0.01	-0.39	0.29	0.67
Hispanic	1.04	0.26	2.84**	0.85	0.27	2.34**	-0.38	0.28	1.83	-0.39	0.20	0.67
Followed H1N1	0.66	0.18	1.93**				0.66	0.27	1.95**			
Interest				1.21	0.18	3.36***				1.14	0.19	3.14**
Constant	-1.76	0.48	0.17**	-1.65	0.48	0.19***	-0.65	0.42	0.52	-0.96	0.44	0.38*
Chi square	80.55**			112.71**			59.24			91.107**		
Nagelke Rsquare	0.13			0.21			0.11			0.17		

[1]Omitted category is less or high school. [2]Omitted category is children under 6. [3]Omitted category is low income. [4]Omitted category is White.
*p < 0.05, **p < 0.01.

We conducted a similar analysis for August 2009. The results for both models are similar, despite the decrease over the months in the levels of following and interest in H1N1 (Table 1). In model 1 the odds ratio for 'Followed' was 1.95 (p < 0.01). In Model 2, the odds ratio for 'Interest' was 3.14 (p < 0.01). In each model the general perception of worry was significantly related to the independent variable with the others controlled. By August 2009 only the age, sex, and marital status variables remained significant in relationship to worry with the independent variables controlled.

Concluding remarks

Our purpose in this study was to explore the relationship of media coverage to fear or worry over infection from the H1N1 in the US during the pandemic of 2009. Consistent with the media agenda-setting framework, our findings show that, beyond social category membership, the extent to which people are interested in the news about the outbreak and followed it closely is correlated with worry. The data are cross sectional and that does not permit a conclusive picture of causation. Is it the media's coverage that stimulates interest and worry, or is it interest and worry that result in greater consumption of media messages? Most likely it is an iterative process in which the media alert people to the outbreak and growth of a pandemic followed by a growing worry or fear of infection on the part of some individuals which leads to even greater attention to the media. At least at the early stages, more than half of the respondents did not develop a worried outlook. Was that because the infection lasted only one flu season? Or was it the result of knowledge of the earlier SARS outbreak that simply bypassed the United States and thus desensitised the population to the threat of a serious flu? Our data do not permit us to undertake answers to these questions. But, they are worth future investigation.

Finally, the findings show that certain social categories – age, sex, and marital status – maintained worry over the possibility of infection beyond their general interest level and the extent to which they followed H1N1 in the news. This probably relates to roles, experiences, and information received through informal social networks. These factors are also worthy of further investigation.

The general limitation of the study is that our two samples are independent. Had they consisted of the same people interviewed at both times we could have pursued the question as to individuals increasing or decreasing in worry as the outbreak continued. Yet, the findings of this exploratory study suggest the central role of media exposure. Even when interest in media reporting decreases, people's concern with infection remains high. Finally, media interest is the most important variable predicting worry with exposure when sociodemographic variables are controlled.

References

Alcabes, P. (2009) *Dread: How Fear and Fantasy Have Fueled Epidemics from the Black Death to the Avian Flu.* New York: Public Affairs Books.

Altheide, D. and Michalowski, R. (1999) Fear in the news: A discourse of control, *The Sociological Quarterly*, 40, 3, 475–503.

Becker, M. (ed.) (1974) *The Health Belief Model and Personal Health Behavior.* San Francisco, CA: Society for Public Health Education, Inc.

Bomlitz, L. and Brezis, M. (2008) Misrepresentation of health risks by mass media, *Journal of Public Health*, 30, 2: 202–4.

Dearing, J. and Rogers, E. (1996) *Agenda Setting*. Thousand Oaks, CA: Sage.

Mesch, G. Schwirian, K.P. and Kolovov, T. (2011) Media coverage and worry over becoming infected: the case of the Swine Flu epidemic of 2009–2010. Presented at the Annual Meeting of the North Central Sociological Association, 2 April 2011, Cleveland, OH.

Rosenstock, I. (1960) Why people use health services, *Milbank Memorial Fund Quarterly*, 44, 3, 94–7.

Shrum, L.J. (2007) The implications of survey method for measuring cultivation effects, *Human Communication Research*, 33, 1, 64–80.

Setbon, M. and Raude, J. (2010) The 2009 pandemic H1N1 influenza vaccination in France: Who accepted to receive the vaccine and why? *European Journal of Public Health*, 20, 5, 490–4.

Warr, M. and Ellison, C.G. (2010) Rethinking social reactions to crime: Personal and altruistic fear in family households, *American Journal of Sociology*, 106, 3, 1033–43.

15

Why the French did not choose to panic: a dynamic analysis of the public response to the influenza pandemic
William Sherlaw and Jocelyn Raude

Introduction

This chapter focuses on the dynamics of risk representations and their potential impact on precautionary behaviour in relation to pandemic influenza among French adults. During the last decade pandemic influenza has received considerable attention from the scientific, political and lay communities worldwide. Prior to the emergence of so-called 'swine flu' in North America, the increasing magnitude of avian influenza outbreaks had raised the spectre of a new and potentially devastating influenza pandemic with consequences comparable to those of Spanish flu (1918–1919). Major public concern was expressed that the current highly pathogenic avian influenza viruses might mutate into more highly infectious forms and acquire the ability of person to person transmission. Such concern was not surprising since pandemic influenza involved most of the properties that have been consistently found to contribute to large media coverage, strong institutional attention and high perceptions of risk (Renn and Rohrmann 2000, Slovic 2000). Indeed, the disease caused by an invisible, unfamiliar, communicable, potentially catastrophic, emerging infectious agent remains at least partly beyond individual and social control due to the extreme difficulty of detecting it before the first symptoms appear.

In the spring of 2009 the spread of a novel A/H1N1 influenza virus triggered the worldwide implementation of mitigating responses planned by public health organisations. Roughly, two major phases may be identified: (i) in the absence of available vaccine, the public was strongly encouraged to adopt a range of preventive behaviour including hygiene and social-distancing measures and (ii) once the vaccine was released, it was recommended that members of high-priority groups, then the population as a whole, should be immunised against the virus at ad hoc vaccination centres. However, in France, as in many western countries, the public health authorities failed to convince a large proportion of the public to undertake health protective behaviour. On the basis of their local experience, many authors have argued in both the lay and scientific media, including prestigious biomedical journals, that this novel influenza pandemic triggered public panic in many developed countries (Bonneux and Van Damme 2010, Gilman 2010). Although there is still no agreement on the objective criteria that accurately define the pattern of collective behaviour that may qualify as a panic, this generally refers to 'an explosion of public concern about a problem – typically unconnected with any sudden change in the underlying risk – followed

Pandemics and Emerging Infectious Diseases: The Sociological Agenda, First Edition. Edited by Robert Dingwall, Lily M. Hoffman and Karen Staniland. Chapters © 2013 The Authors. Book Compilation © 2013 Foundation for the Sociology of Health & Illness / John Wiley & Sons Ltd.

by an also sudden collapse of concern' (Loewenstein *et al.* 2001: 278). Danielle Ofri also alleged in the *New England Journal of Medicine* that 'the dramatic shift in public sentiment over the course of this A/H1N1 epidemic . . . bears only a faint connection to the actual disease epidemiology of the virus' (2009: 2595). However, to date little, if any, empirical evidence has been provided to support the assumption that there was a panic. Indeed, the few studies to collect longitudinal data during the pandemic tend to demonstrate, to the contrary, that the level of fear or anxiety expressed by laypeople remained very moderate over time (Rubin *et al.* 2010, Gidengil *et al.* 2012).

In line with influenza preparedness planning, the French government ordered approximately 60,000,000 doses of vaccine so that 75 per cent of the population might receive two doses. Given that the vaccine took several months to become available, a prioritisation plan was announced in which the most vulnerable (the chronically sick, healthcare staff and parents of young infants) were given the opportunity to get vaccinated for free. The potential benefits for these groups were threefold: personal protection, protection of their relatives and reduced absenteeism. Nevertheless, vaccination was rapidly extended to the rest of the population as there was good evidence the vaccine was very effective in preventing serologically confirmed influenza, and had limited side-effects. Despite this, the influenza vaccine uptake among the French remained low: constituting only nine per cent of the population by January 2010. This low vaccination rate reminds us that the failure or success of any prevention programme is ultimately determined by how the public thinks about and evaluates health threats, as well as the effectiveness of mitigating measures promoted by the health authorities.

Empirical data and theoretical constructs have been employed to explain why a large majority of French people rejected the pandemic influenza vaccine. Indeed, the relative inefficacy of the influenza prevention programme raises several crucial questions: how did the representations of the pandemic threat evolve over this period, affecting decisions to engage in protective health behaviour such as vaccination? How was the pandemic threat framed in the scientific and lay press prior to the emergence of the virus? And, given that pandemic threat presented virtually all the characteristics consistently found to elicit high concern and intensive media coverage (it was unknown, new, insidious, catastrophic, invisible and so on), why did most people eventually not panic? Our analysis of the public's response to the 2009 influenza pandemic incorporates: (i) findings from a series of surveys carried out at different stages of the epidemic, (ii) scrutiny of French mass media and international scientific press and (iii) insights from theoretical frameworks related to a sequence analysis approach such as innovation diffusion theory, surprise theory and social representation theory.

Sequence analysis of health behaviour during the influenza pandemic

The dynamic and context of health-related behaviour – including beliefs, attitudes and feelings – during the influenza pandemic may be investigated through complementary theoretical frameworks that may be usefully classified as belonging to a sequence analysis approach. The main assumption of this important approach is that actions or events cannot be analysed separately from their temporal context. According to Abbott (1995: 94), emphasising context means basically that one should be less willing to think about cases independent of one another, and often from the past. Indeed, sociologists and psychologists have noted that a large range of health and social behaviours seem to develop in orderly sequence. As pointed out by Howard Becker in his famous study of *Outsiders* (1966: 23):

we must deal with a sequence of steps, of changes in the individual's behaviors and perspectives in order to understand the phenomenon. Each step requires explanation, and what may operate at one step in the sequence may be of negligible importance at another step.

In the last decades a considerable number of conceptual and methodological instruments have been developed to promote sequence analysis in the social and behavioural sciences (Abbott 2001). However, to date, with a few rare exceptions, most authors have chosen to ignore the sequence aspects in their investigations of health protective behaviour in response to the 2009 influenza pandemic threat.

Nonetheless, this remains relatively surprising since social and behavioural sciences related to health issues are characterised by a long tradition of sequential research. Thus, in health economics, several authors investigating safety crises have shown that the formation and updating of health protective behaviour may function as a stochastic process, in which the precaution taken at time $t + 1$ are to a large extent determined by the precautions taken at time t, and so forth. In health psychology a set of sequential models called stage theories – such as Diclemente's transtheoretical model or Weinstein's precaution adoption process model – have been proposed in the literature from the late 1970s. These models have been developed in opposition to classical motivational models – derived from the rational choice theory – that essentially focus on the probabilistic and consequential factors underpinning health-related behaviour at one point in time (Armitage and Conner 2000). The sequential models assume that decision-making in relation to the adoption of precautionary behaviour fundamentally consists of moving through distinct stages. One notable exception aimed at improving cross-sectional analysis may be found in studies treating vaccination campaigns as examples of diffusion of preventive innovations.

Complementing the sequential approach, certain sociologists such as Rogers (1995) have studied the social process of diffusion of innovations, which may be defined as 'an idea, knowledge, a belief or social norm, a product or service, a technology or process . . . as long as it is perceived to be new' (Dearing and Meyer 2006: 34). Diffusion theory may be applied to any material or social good provided one can identify suitable indicators of diffusion and it thus has a wide application to health and illness issues. This includes health promotion and public health prevention plans aimed at reducing unhealthy behaviour, and vaccination. Diffusion depends on many different factors associated with the characteristics of the innovation (like simplicity, effectiveness and compatibility) and on the characteristics of the population in which the diffusion takes place, as well as the source of the innovation and the characteristics of the diffuser. As Valente and Myers (2010) have memorably stated, 'the messenger is the medium'. This may be particularly relevant to vaccination. Diffusion theory is applicable to any diffusible good and offers valuable insights into the acceptance or non-acceptance of vaccination. When one maps the percentage of people within a population taking up an innovation against time a typical S-shaped curve emerges. The individuals in the population may be divided into categories according to time of adoption. Within this ideal schema we may typically speak of innovators, early adopters, early majority, late majority or laggards (Rogers 1995). These categories correspond to extensive empirical evidence in quantitative terms. Nevertheless, they reveal the positivist and normative nature of the approach. There is an assumption that (i) the innovation is valued, (ii) that people should take it up and (iii) that the diffusers should do all in their power to achieve this goal. Arguably these assumptions may be questioned in the case of innovations in general and in public health and vaccination in particular.

Several authors have mobilised diffusion science to improve vaccination rates or understand preventive attitudes (Agyeman *et al.* 2009, Britto *et al.* 2006, 2007, Freed *et al.* 1998, Nougairède *et al.* 2010). Although it is difficult to argue that influenza A/H1N1 vaccination per se is innovative since vaccination, campaigns and immunisation have a long history, going back to Lady Montagu and smallpox inoculation, nevertheless the attempt by public health officials and governments throughout the world to orchestrate true mass vaccination using little tested vaccines against influenza in a race against the clock, under the full exposure of the media, may be considered innovative. In considering the uptake of a vaccine by the population there is a tendency to restrict the application of the theory to the vaccine. In the case of the 2009 influenza pandemic another parallel diffusion process must be considered, namely the contagion of the population by the virus itself. This has been well-recognised by Nougairède *et al.* (2010) who have applied diffusion theory to the pandemic in France using both media and serological data.

Diffusion theory becomes increasingly powerful if harnessed in the spirit of sequence analysis to study, not just the diffusion of the vaccine (which should also take into account the diffusion of the disease itself and the status of the organisation implementing the preventive measures) but also the information diffused from different sources about the vaccine and the disease. In such an approach the diffusion of anti-vaccination messages concerning possible side-effects such as Guillain–Barré syndrome as well as messages concerning the innocuousness of the disease may be considered to be in outright competition with the official government campaign for arms and minds. Such matters concern scientific facts and estimates of risks, but also social representation and risk perception as well as trust in public health experts, government ministers and the pharmaceutical industry.

The diffusion of any preventive innovation takes considerable time (Rogers 2002). As Agyeman *et al.* (2009) have pointed out in relation to rotavirus immunisation, it is crucial to make the transition from the early adopters to early majority phase to achieve good coverage. If 50 per cent of a population support an innovation one may generally predict a greater than 80 per cent implementation. In the case of Influenza A/H1N1 was there sufficient time to reach a critical mass to ensure the successful diffusion of the vaccine to the population? This remains an interesting question to address in future work. During the 2009 French pandemic many classic vaccinology concerns known since the eighteenth century (Rusnock 2002) came to the fore, such as the severity of the disease, the relative risk of getting vaccinated and the weighing up of health gains and losses, especially between present and future risks, for the individual, family and community. Questions on conflicts of interest over the vaccine also featured in the media. In the weeks prior to the vaccine well-known public health figures offered competing views on the seriousness of the disease and the appropriateness of the costly measures. Although this cocktail of issues necessarily framed the vaccination campaign we suggest that when the vaccine became available the public, as lay epidemiologists, tended to trust the evidence of their own eyes rather than previous alarming estimates of morbidity and death offered by experts, with consequent effects on vaccine uptake.

Two other complementary frameworks related to sequence analysis cast light on the influenza pandemic, especially in relation to actual or intended vaccination. First, in line with Shackle's surprise theory small but significant changes in the distribution of perceived risk may potentially have elicited more substantial behavioural modification than the absolute level of perceived risk. Secondly, we will show that anchoring, as conceptualised by Moscovici's social representations theory, provides an insightful framework to reveal a sequence that may partially explain the mild reaction of the public to 2009 A/H1N1 influenza pandemic health risk.

Effects of perceptions on health behaviour during the pandemic: state or change?

Many empirical investigations have been devoted to understand health behaviour in response to the 2009 global influenza pandemic. Given the efforts of the scientific community, one would have expected that causes of health protective behaviour were now relatively well identified and understood. But, surprisingly, this is not the case: the variance of health protective behaviour explained by conventional social and cognitive factors is typically small, and their effect on actual behaviour or even behavioural intentions remains weak despite their statistical significance. This may be due to the basically non-sequential character of the methodologies used in most of these studies. Notably, Weinstein has shown in a series of articles that cross-sectional research designs are not well adapted to demonstrating the causal relation between a particular construct and health behaviour, partly because these designs implicitly assume that a shift from inaction to action is 'adequately explained by quantitative differences in the value of the decision equation' (Weinstein 1988: 358). Currently, there is still no agreement among social scientists as to whether one should favour temporal changes or distributions at one point of time in the value of independent variables tested to predict health behaviour (Loewenstein and Mather 1990).

Among the possible causes of health behaviour, individuals' risk perceptions have undoubtedly been the most frequently investigated variable. This is not surprising, since risk-related judgments are a central construct in most agent-based theories of health behaviour (Gochman 1997). In the past decade it has been found that perceived risks are consistently and significantly associated with the likelihood of taking a range of preventive actions to cope with health threats, in particular to get vaccinated against seasonal influenza (Brewer *et al.* 2007). Risk perception commonly refers to intuitive judgments that people make on being asked in a variety of ways to evaluate hazardous activities (Slovic 2000). Although several competing conceptualisations of this construct have been offered since the late 1970s, there is relative agreement that perceived risk can be defined as the combination of two key dimensions: the perceived likelihood of harm and the perceived severity of the consequences. These components are assumed to motivate people to protect themselves from health risks.

Recently, a third core dimension has been incorporated into this concept: the affective response to health risk (such as fear or anxiety). There is increasing empirical evidence that affective variables are better predictors of health protective behaviour than the purely cognitive and probabilistic judgements related to risk (Chapman and Coups 2006, Loewenstein *et al.* 2001, Weinstein *et al.* 2007).

However, the hypothesis according to which preventive action or inaction in response to an influenza pandemic may result from the difference in perceptions before and after the event remains poorly investigated in the current literature. Informed by pioneering research in the domain of health behaviour (Loewenstein and Mather 1990), we have come to the view that surprise may play a crucial role in the public response to a health threat. In the social and cognitive sciences, surprise is commonly defined as an outcome of the distance between the distributions of beliefs of the observers before and after. In other words, 'Surprise occurs when events deviate from prior expectations' (Loewenstein and Mather 1990: 169). To date, it has been widely demonstrated that the greater the distance between posterior and prior distributions of beliefs endorsed by subjects, the stronger the response to the event in terms of adaptation, learning, attention or emotion (Itti and Baldi 2009, Baldi and Itti 2010).

Ideally, a rigorous testing of this hypothesis would require the collection of data for the same group of individuals before and after the emergence of the so-called swine flu within a longitudinal research design (Loewenstein 1990). As such panel data do not exist (even if a small number of longitudinal studies have been carried out after the emergence of the disease), we more modestly use aggregated data that have been collected in cross-sectional surveys devoted to the perceived risk associated with pandemic influenza at different key points in time. This research presents the advantage of having employed consistent question wording and sampling procedures in three different surveys. It should be noted, neverthe-less, that this methodology may be prone to small but significant biases in the interpretation of research results (Weinstein *et al.* 2007).

Data were collected by telephone from representative samples of the adult population through three cross-sectional studies; in June 2008, June 2009 and December 2009. These correspond to three critical points in time related to the epidemic in France: (i) one year before the emergence of the 2009 A/H1N1 epidemic, (ii) the period immediately following the epidemiological observation of the first indigenous cases of 2009 A/H1N1 pandemic influenza, and (iii) one month after the launch of vaccination. For each survey the sample ($N = 1000$) was selected by computer-generated random digit dialling and stratified accord-ing to gender, age group, occupation and geographical area. The three above-mentioned measures of risk perception – perceived severity, vulnerability and anxiety – were repeatedly assessed on the basis of questions employing a similar wording derived from the existing literature (de Zwart *et al.* 2007) by using either a scale of 0–10 or one of 0–100.[1] Mean scores related to these three variables are reported for each point of the time in Table 1. ANOVA showed that these mean scores were all statistically different over time. A series of six Student's *t* tests were also performed on each pair of the same variable at the different points in time, using $P < 0.001$ as a criterion for significance. All the pairings were found to be significantly different except anxiety in wave 2 versus anxiety in wave 3.

Paradoxically, these temporal data tend to demonstrate that all the dimensions of the perceived risk associated with infection significantly decreased just after the emergence of the 2009 A/H1N1 influenza epidemic in France, giving credence to the surprise effect. The perceived severity of the disease continued to decrease during the pandemic while the per-ceived vulnerability was found to rise above the level of spring 2008. Interestingly, the level of anxiety seems to have remained relatively constant during the epidemic. This may be largely attributed to the contradictory trends that distinguished between the pandemic's perceived severity and people's vulnerability over time. Overall, the dynamic pattern of risk perceptions identified in France do not give empirical support to the hypothesis of a public panic in the sense of a temporary but strong surge of concern in the general population as a whole, even when there was no evidence of change in the underlying risks. These results are relatively congruent with those obtained from a number of cross-sectional and longitu-dinal studies performed after the emergence of the 2009 A/H1N1 influenza pandemic

Table 1 *Measures of risk perception over time: means and standard deviations in parentheses*

Variable	June 2008	June 2009	Dec. 2009	F-value	P-value
Perceived vulnerability (0–100)	28.68 (25.42)	19.53 (19.43)	39.80 (21.17)	195.82	0.000
Perceived severity (0–10)	6.71 (2.25)	5.85 (2.38)	5.16 (1.92)	121.19	0.000
Expressed anxiety (0–10)	5.03 (2.90)	4.03 (2.63)	4.16 (2.31)	42.60	0.000
Observations (*n*)	1003	1001	1003		

throughout the world, showing a mild emotional and behavioural response to the risk of infection at the early stage of the pandemic, which steadily declined over time.

Sequence analysis offers a very convincing though insufficient explanation of this relative apathy, which can be related to the effect of disconfirmed expectations. As could have been postulated a priori from surprise theory, epidemiological outcomes that fall below expectations tend to generate a feeling of relief, while those that are above expectations favour the formation of a panic, which is often viewed as the exaggerated reaction to an emerging threat. Nevertheless, these empirical data raise a crucial question. Why did many people expect potentially catastrophic and frightening consequences due to the emergence of a novel pandemic influenza virus? In other words, where did these pre-pandemic expectations of high risk come from? As outlined by many social scientists, one should not consider that ideas about risk are independent variables (Joffe 2003). What, then, were the framing effects that may have shaped the content of social representations related to the 2009 influenza pandemic?

The 1918 Spanish flu: an anchor for the future influenza pandemic?

Lay epidemiology focuses on the framing of health and illness and refers to schemes:

> in which individuals interpret health risks through the routine observation and discussion of cases of illness and death in their personal networks and in the public arena, as well as from formal and informal evidence arising from other sources, such as television and magazines. (Frankel *et al.* 1991: 428)

Such framing involves a socio-cognitive process of selecting and interpreting information relied on to understand and respond to an event or issue. It is increasingly recognised that people's knowledge of the world – including health threats – comes from perceptual and symbolic representations conveyed by the audio-visual and newsprint media. Mass media thus tend to frame our representations of the world in particular ways, by making some information more salient than other information (Kuypers 2002: 18).

The anchoring process derived from Moscovici's social representations theory is one of the best documented framing effects on media coverage and social recognition of emerging infectious diseases, such as acquired immune deficiency syndrome, severe acute respiratory syndrome (SARS) or Creutzfeldt–Jakob disease epidemics (Joffe 1996, Washer 2004, 2006). Anchoring consists of a series of social cognitive transformations by which people acquire, classify, label and recall unfamiliar issues or events on the basis of an existing order of things that is meaningful for them (Moscovici 2001). As Zerubavel notes (1999: 24), in order to make sense of novel situations we thus try to mentally force them into pre-existing schemas. Empirical social representations research has demonstrated that risk events are rarely recognised and thought of separately from their historical and cultural context. However, Joffe (2003: 63) notes that meaning is made of many newly discovered mass illnesses in line with those known, whatever their differences at a material level. Interestingly, this often leads to the transfer of illegitimate properties from past to current health threats. People are willing to attribute to a new epidemiological event a range of features that may no longer be accurate or relevant to it.

Several recent studies have shown that prior to the emergence of the swine flu in North America, the imminent threat of a pandemic was frequently linked to the 1918 influenza pandemic. In the UK Nerlich and Halliday (2007: 61) found in the national press a strong pattern of reference to previous flu pandemics, in particular to the so-called Spanish Influenza of 1918. They also argued that this metaphorical framing elicited alarmist expectations in relation to the infectious risk. Similarly, Abeysinghe and White (2010: 369) showed the existence of historical continuity in the construction of epidemics in Australian society through the link between avian influenza and the Spanish flu pandemic of 1918. Informed by this previous work, we have tested the hypothesis that the 1918 Spanish flu served as a historical reference in the French media coverage of the 2009 influenza pandemic.

Four types of source (see Table 2) were used to examine the dynamics of media coverage of the 1918 Spanish flu over time in France. The media reviewed included the scientific press (through academic journals referenced in the ISI Web of Knowledge database), the national news, radio and television coverage (through channels surveyed by the French National Audio-visual Institute), and national newspapers (through online archives). Since the main purpose of this analysis was not to describe the content of the media coverage but to study whether the Spanish flu may have served as a historical anchor for the forthcoming (2009) influenza pandemic, only two newspapers of different political persuasions were chosen: the left-oriented *Le Monde* and the conservative *Le Figaro*. The corpus comprised all items – either articles or programmes – that contained the words 'Spanish flu' or 'Spanish influenza' in the reviewed period. As indicated in Table 2, the choice of the period was essentially pragmatic: items were all available online from existing databases, with the exception of the scientific articles for which we arbitrarily started the analysis in 1980. However, only five articles mentioning the 1918 Spanish flu in their abstracts were found between 1920 and 1980. As illustrated in Figure 1, these three different measures of media coverage were highly correlated ($r > .5$, $P < 0.001$), in particular newspapers and audiovisual media ($r > .9$, $P < 0.001$), and similar trends were observed over time.

A brief analysis of the media coverage of the Spanish flu shows that this major epidemiological phenomenon remained of interest to a number of historians until the mid-1990s. In the last decade the SARS epidemic, followed by several H5N1 avian influenza outbreaks in Asia, seems to have revived the collective memory of the dramatic Spanish flu event. Indeed, the rapid rise in the number of media reports mentioning Spanish Influenza demonstrate that biomedical scientists and journalists used this event as an anchor, contributing to framing the social representations of the forthcoming pandemic threat not as an ordinary infectious respiratory disease but rather as a form of modern plague. Even if it is clear that media treatment cannot determine how members of the public actually think about the risk (Joffe 2011), this was later interpreted as an attempt to mobilise people by arousing fear and exaggerating the seriousness of the threat. Paradoxically, the choice of this alarmist anchor may have been highly counterproductive: rather than rendering the pandemic influenza more threatening, once the first cases of infection had been observed, it elicited a

Table 2 *Characteristics of the media reviewed*

Type of media	Period	Databases	Number of items found
Scientific press	1980–2010	ISI Web of Knowledge	373 articles
National newspapers	1987–2010	Archives of *Le Monde* and *Le Figaro*	189 articles
National TV	1989–2010	Archives of the French National Audio-visual Institute	69 programmes
National radio	1989–2010	Archives of the French National Audio-visual Institute	53 programmes

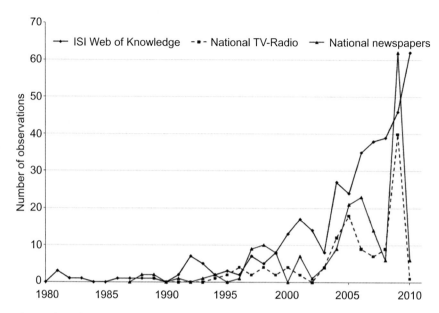

Figure 1 *Number of articles or programmes in the media that mention Spanish flu*

relative indifference to the health authorities' promotion of pharmaceutical and non-pharmaceutical interventions. By summer 2009 the anchor was seen to change suddenly from Spanish flu to a so-called *grippette* (chill) – a term coined by a well-known French politician and medical expert – in the non-scientific media. Symbolising the actual lessening of fear and perceived seriousness, this shift may be partly attributed to the fact that the pattern of morbidity and mortality identified at this time was more like that of seasonal influenza epidemics than the historical pandemic of 1918 (Raude *et al*. 2010).

Conclusion

Emerging infectious diseases have consistently been found to be prone to arousing panic, or what has also been called the 'social amplification of risk' (Kasperson *et al*. 2001). Most authors attribute this propensity to the fact that this category of events combines several key factors that are known to attract attention from the media, populations and institutions (Kasperson *et al*. 2001, Slovic 2000, Smith 2006). Paradoxically, as pointed out previously, the emergence of the 2009 A/H1N1 pandemic influenza does not seem to have triggered panic, even if a range of behavioural changes in response to the threat has been reported in the literature. This is exemplified by the relative failure of the vaccination campaign in France, as in most surveyed countries. Why then did people not panic when faced with the actual threat of infection from pandemic influenza?

In relation to the study of emerging infectious diseases (EID) in general and the A/H1N1 pandemic, a number of different explanations have been advanced to explain the low public response, as evinced by low vaccination rates. Notably, Joffe (2011: 457) suggests that we may be seeing evidence of a growing reflexivity in modern societies associated with EID fatigue 'that is reshaping aspects of the social representation of EID in the West'. While this may well be a part of the explanation, recent crises such as the 2011 outbreak of

Escherichia Coli in Germany do not seem to confirm this trend (Paterson 2011). Moreover, in line with our French data, the available longitudinal data collected in the UK (Rubin *et al.* 2010) and in the USA (Gidengil *et al.* 2012) note that the levels of anxiety or the intention to be vaccinated began to fall long before the emergence of controversies around potential conflicts of interests or the safety of the vaccine.

Sequence analysis suggests that this relatively calm attitude may be typically attributed to the positive surprise generated by the gap between people's epidemiological expectations and their observation of the actual illness. Thus, our data tend, surprisingly, to give empirical support to the World Health Organisation (WHO) Director Margaret Chan's comments on the WHO's management of the pandemic threat, that 'part of the problem arises from the big difference between what was expected, after watching the highly lethal H5N1 virus for so long, and what fortunately happened' (Chan 2010). As indicated above, these expectations may be linked to the alarmist framing of the pandemic threat based on frightening metaphors or historical events. The recurrent reference to the 1918 Spanish flu by biomedical scientists and journalists generated representations of the future event in order to try and affect social and political actions in the present (Nerlich and Halliday 2007: 50). Surprise effects related to anchoring may potentially have enormous consequences on the allocation (or misallocation) of human and material resources devoted to public health.

Rubin *et al.* (2010) suggested that increasing levels of anxiety may lead to a higher uptake of behavioural recommendations, including vaccination. But they rightly point out the double-edged nature of attempts to heighten population awareness of an emerging health threat cloaked in uncertainty. There is a thin line between preparedness and alarmism. In relation to the 2009 A/H1N1 influenza pandemic episode the positive metaphor of a rehearsal has often been evoked, but from the public's perspective, it may be that the rehearsal and framing bequeathed by the epidemic has left us with a more problematic legacy. The general lesson to draw from a sequence analysis approach is that our treatment of previous public health crises will inevitably set the stage for tackling future emerging threats. Response to public health threats should be seen in context as involving a social learning process. Consequently, an evidence-based policy is called for to allow the public response to match the severity of the emergent threat and to avoid the risk of undermining public trust. More specifically, it is likely that the framing of the 2009 A/H1N1 event, rather than rehearsing the public to better face future EID threats, may have undermined trust and thereby reduced our capacity to mobilise the public in the case of less benign health threats.

Note

1   Measurement details for each survey have been published separately elsewhere (Raude and Setbon 2009, Setbon *et al.* 2011).

References

Abbott, A. (1995) Sequence-analysis: new methods for old ideas, *Annual Review of Sociology*, 21, 93–113.
Abbott, A. (2001) *Time Matters: On Theory and Method*. Chicago: University of Chicago Press.
Abeysinghe, S. and White, K. (2010) Framing disease: the avian influenza pandemic in Australia, *Health Sociology Review*, 19, 3, 369–81.

Agyeman, P., Desgrandchamps, D., Vaudaux, B., *et al.* (2009) Interpretation of primary care physicians' attitude regarding rotavirus immunisation using diffusion of innovation theories, *Vaccine*, 27, 35, 4771–5.

Armitage, C.J. and Conner, M. (2000) Social cognition models and health behaviour: a structured review, *Psychology and Health*, 15, 173–89.

Baldi, P.F. and Itti, L. (2010) Of bits and wows: a Bayesian theory of surprise with applications to attention, *Neural Networks*, 23, 5, 649–66.

Becker, H.S. (1966) *Outsiders: Studies in the Sociology of Deviance.* New York: Free Press.

Bonneux, L. and Van Damme, W. (2010) Preventing iatrogenic pandemics of panic. Do it in a NICE way? *BMJ*, 340, 3065.

Brewer, N.T., Chapman, G.B., Gibbons, F.X., Gerrard, M., McCaul, K.D. and Weinstein, N.D. (2007) Meta-analysis of the relationship between risk perception and health behavior: the example of vaccination, *Health Psychology*, 26, 2, 136–45.

Britto, M.T., Pandzik, C.G., Meeks, M.S. and Kotagal, U.R. (2006) Combining evidence and diffusion of innovation theory to enhance influenza immunization, *Joint Commission Journal on Quality and Patient Safety*, 32, 8, 426–32.

Britto, M.T., Schoettker, P.J., Pandzik, G.M., Weiland, J., *et al.* (2007) Improving influenza immunisation for high-risk children and adolescents, *Quality and Safety in Health Care*, 16, 5, 363–8.

Chan, M. (2010) Progress in public health during the previous decade and major challenges ahead. Report by the Director-General to the Executive Board at its 126th session, Geneva: 18 January.

Chapman, G.B. and Coups, E.J. (2006) Emotions and preventive health behavior: worry, regret, and influenza vaccination, *Health Psychology*, 25, 1, 82–90.

de Zwart, O., Veldhuijzen, I.K., Elam, G., Aro, A.R., *et al.* (2007) Avian influenza risk perception, Europe and Asia, *Emerging Infectious Diseases*, 13, 2, 290–3.

Dearing, J.W. and Meyer, G. (2006) Revisiting diffusion theory. In Singhal, A. and Dearing, J.W. (eds) *Communication of Innovations.* London: Sage.

Frankel, S., Davison, C. and Smith, G.D. (1991) Lay epidemiology and the rationality of responses to health education, *British Journal of General Practice*, 41, 428–30.

Freed, G.L., Pathman, D.E., Konrad, T.R., Freeman, V.A., *et al.* (1998) Adopting immunization recommendations: a new dissemination model, *Maternal Child Health*, 2, 4, 231–9.

Gidengil, C.A., Parker, A.M. and Zikmund-Fisher, B.J. (2012) Trends in risk perceptions and vaccination intentions: a longitudinal study of the first year of the H1N1 pandemic, *American Journal of Public Health*, 102, 4, 672–9.

Gilman, S.L. (2010) Moral panic and pandemics, *Lancet*, 375, 9729, 1866–7.

Gochman, D.S. (1997) *Handbook of Health Behavior Research I: Personal and Social Determinants.* New York: Plenum Press.

Itti, L. and Baldi, P.F. (2009) Bayesian surprise attracts human attention, *Vision Research*, 49, 10, 1295–306.

Joffe, H. (1996) AIDS research and prevention: a social representational approach, *British Journal of Medical Psychology*, 69, 3, 169–90.

Joffe, H. (2003) Risk: from perception to social representation, *British Journal of Social Psychology*, 42, 1, 55–73.

Joffe, H. (2011) Public apprehension of emerging infectious diseases: are changes afoot? *Public Understanding of Science*, 20, 4, 446–60.

Kasperson, R.E., Jhaveri, N. and Kasperson, J.X. (2001) Stigma and the social amplification of risk: toward a frame-work of analysis. In Flynn J., Slovic P. and Kunreuther K. (eds) *Risk, Media and Stigma: Understanding Public Challenges to Modern Science and Technology.* London: Earthscan.

Kuypers, A. (2002) *Press Bias and Politics: How the Media Frame Controversial Issues.* Westport: Greenwood.

Loewenstein, G. and Mather, J. (1990) Dynamic processes in risk perception, *Journal of Risk and Uncertainty*, 3, 2, 155–75.

Loewenstein, G.F., Weber, E.U., Hsee, C.K. and Welch, N. (2001) Risk as feelings, *Psychological Bulletin*, 127, 2, 267–86.

Moscovici, S. (2001) *Social Representations.* New York: University Press.

Nerlich, B. and Halliday, C. (2007) Avian flu: the creation of expectations in the interplay between science and the media, *Sociology of Health and Illness*, 29, 1, 46–65.

Nougairède, A., Lagier, J.C., Ninove, L., Sartor, C., *et al.* (2010) Likely correlation between sources of information and acceptability of A/H1N1 swine-origin influenza virus vaccine in Marseille, France, *PLoS ONE*, 5, 6, e11292. J; doi:10.1371/journal.pone.0011292.

Ofri, D. (2009) The emotional epidemiology of H1N1 influenza vaccination, *New England Journal of Medicine*, 361, 27, 2594–5.

Paterson, T. (2011) E. coli: panic grips Germany while Britain waits nervously, *The Independent*, 4 June, available at http://www.independent.co.uk/life-style/health-and-families/health-news/ecoli-panic-grips-germany-while-britain-waits-nervously-2292889.html (accessed 15 August 2012).

Raude, J. and Setbon, M. (2009) Lay perceptions of the pandemic influenza threat, *European Journal of Epidemiology*, 24, 7, 339–42.

Raude, J., Caille-Brillet, A.L. and Setbon, M. (2010) The 2009 pandemic H1N1 influenza vaccination in France: who accepted to receive the vaccine and why? *PLoS Currents Influenza*, available at http://www.ncbi.nlm.nih.gov/pmc/articles/PMC2957695/?tool=pubmed (accessed 15 August 2012).

Renn, O. and Rohrmann, B. (2000) *Cross-Cultural Risk Perception: a Survey of Empirical Studies*. Dordrecht: Kluwer Academic.

Rogers, E.M. (1995) *Diffusion of Innovations*. New York: Free Press.

Rogers, E.M. (2002) Diffusion of preventive innovations, *Addictive Behaviours*, 27, 6, 989–93.

Rubin, G., Potts, H. and Michie, S. (2010) the impact of communications about swine flu (influenza A H1N1v) on public responses to the outbreak: results from 36 national telephone surveys in the UK, *Health Technology Assessment*, 14, 34, 183–266.

Rusnock, A.A. (2002) *Vital Accounts: Quantifying Health and Population in Eighteenth Century England and France*. Cambridge: Cambridge University Press.

Setbon, M., Le Pape, M.C., Letroublon, C, Caille-Brillet, A.L., *et al.* (2011) The public's preventive strategies in response to the pandemic influenza A/H1N1 in France: distribution and determinants, *Preventive Medicine*, 52, 2, 178–81.

Slovic, P. (2000) *The Perception of Risk*. Earthscan: London.

Smith, R.D. (2006) Responding to global infectious disease outbreaks: lessons from SARS on the role of risk perception, communication and management, *Social Sciences and Medicine*, 63, 12, 3113–23.

Valente, T.W. and Myers, R. (2010) The messenger is the medium: communication and diffusion principles in the process of behavior change, *Estudios sobre las Culturas Contemporáneas Época II*, 16, 31, 249–76.

Washer, P. (2006) Representations of mad cow disease, *Social Sciences and Medicine*, 62, 2, 457–66.

Washer, P. (2004) Representations of SARS in the British newspapers, *Social Science and Medicine*, 59, 12, 2561–71.

Weinstein, N. (1988) The precaution adoption process, *Health Psychology*, 7, 4, 355–86.

Weinstein, N.D., Kwitel, A., McCaul, K.D., Magnan, R.E., *et al.* (2007) Risk perceptions: assessment and relationship to influenza vaccination, *Health Psychology*, 26, 2, 146–51.

Zerubavel, E. (1999) *Social Mindscapes: An Invitation to Cognitive Sociology*. Cambridge: Harvard University Press.

Index

Pandemics and Emerging Infectious Diseases: The Sociological Agenda, First Edition. Edited by
Robert Dingwall, Lily M. Hoffman and Karen Staniland. Chapters © 2013 The Authors. Book
Compilation © 2013 Foundation for the Sociology of Health & Illness / John Wiley & Sons Ltd.